REFLEXOLOGY
for BEGINNERS

Reflexology: The Foot Path to Wellness

Reflexology is a simple, effective method of complementary therapy. By gently massaging specific areas on the sole of the foot, you can treat specific ailments and enhance overall physical, emotional, and mental health.

Reflexology for Beginners includes clear, complete, illustrated instructions. Even if you have no prior knowledge of these methods, you can use them immediately, as you are guided from the basics through a full reflexology session by David Vennells, a qualified and experienced practitioner. The book also includes a fascinating introduction to the history and underlying principles of this energy-cleansing and balancing technique.

Start today on the path to healing as you discover for yourself why reflexology is widely used in many hospitals, hospices, and treatment centers.

About the Author

David F. Vennells is a qualified reflexologist and Reiki teacher. He currently resides and practices in north-west England.

To Write to the Author

If you wish to contact the author or would like more information about this book, please write to the author in care of Llewellyn Worldwide, and we will forward your request. Both the author and publisher appreciate hearing from you. Llewellyn Worldwide cannot guarantee that every letter written to the author can be answered, but all will be forwarded. Please write to:

David F. Vennells
% Llewellyn Worldwide
P.O. Box 64383, 0-7387-0098-3
St. Paul, MN 55164-0383, U.S.A.

Please enclose a self-addressed, stamped envelope for reply, or $1.00 to cover costs. If outside the U.S.A., enclose international postal reply coupon.

Many of Llewellyn's authors have websites with additional information and resources. For more information, please visit our website at
http://www.llewellyn.com

REFLEXOLOGY for BEGINNERS

Healing Through
Foot Massage
of Pressure Points

David F. Vennells

2001
Llewellyn Publications
St. Paul, Minnesota 55164-0383

FIRST EDITION
First printing, 2001

Cover design: Gavin Dayton Duffy
Cover photo: © Victoria Revillas/Superstock
Editing and book design: Christine Snow
Interior illustrations: Mary Ann Zapalac
Medicine Buddha illustration: Courtesy of Tharpa Publications
    © 1990. Illustration by Andy Weber.

Library of Congress Cataloging-in-Publication Data
    Vennells, David F.
        Reflexology for beginners: healing through foot massage of
            pressure points / David F. Vennells.
            p. cm.
        Includes bibliographical references and index.
        ISBN 0-7387-0098-3
        1. Reflexology (Therapy) I. Title.

    RM723.R43 V464 2001
    615.8'22–dc21   2001038688

Llewellyn Publications
A Division of Llewellyn Worldwide, Ltd.
P.O. Box 64383, Dept. 0-7387-0098-3
St. Paul, MN 55164-0383
www.llewellyn.com

Printed in the United States of America

Other Books by David F. Vennells

Reiki for Beginners
(Llewellyn Publications, 1999)

Bach Flower Remedies for Beginners
(Llewellyn Publications, 2001)

Acknowledgments

Sincere thanks to everyone who has contributed to the making of this book.

Special love and thanks to Mum and Dad and all my family and friends.

Thanks also to Simon Duncan at the Association of Reflexologists in the UK for his help and for the good work of the association. Reflexology is in good hands!

Many thanks to the editor, Christine Snow, for another excellent and professional job.

Greatest thanks always to my spiritual guide, who makes all good things possible.

Contents

Illustrations

Author's Note

Any advice given from a Buddhist perspective to support the practice of reflexology is simply what I have found to be helpful from my own experience and from receiving teachings on Buddhism. Any reader interested in deepening his or her knowledge of Buddhism or learning to meditate should consult the information given in appendices 1 and 2.

All reflexology books differ slightly in the exact location of reflex points on the feet. The diagrams in this book show the reflexes as they were taught to me at college, and they are the ones I have found to be most effective.

Editor's Note

The practices and techniques described in this book should not be used as an alternative to professional medical treatment. This book does not attempt to give any medical diagnosis, treatment, prescription, or suggestion for medication in relation to any human disease, pain, injury, deformity, or physical or mental condition.

The author and publisher of this book are not responsible in any manner whatsoever for any injury that may occur through following the instructions contained herein. It is recommended that before beginning any reflexology treatment, you consult your physician to determine whether you are medically, physically, and mentally fit to undertake this course of practice.

Introduction

My first experience of reflexology as a therapy was when I was in my early twenties. I had heard of it before then, but as with most healthy people who do not have a direct interest in health or healing matters, I really had no idea of what was involved. Certainly if I had remained healthy I would not have made an effort to find out more about reflexology, discover its benefits, become a reflexologist, and eventually write this book. It is funny how things work out!

Before I decided to try reflexology I had been very ill for several years with chronic fatigue syndrome (CFS). I spent most of my time lying down or being pushed around in a wheelchair. The medical profession had identified the condition and told me that it was the result of my body not being able to get over a previous bout of glandular fever. However, they were unable to offer any practical help in the form of treatment although a course of anti-depressants did help me when going through a particularly despondent time. Unfortunately I was not warned that following glandular fever the patient should rest completely for up to two months until all symptoms have passed and full strength is regained. If this advice is not followed the sufferer is much more likely to develop long-term postviral fatigue syndrome, as I did.

After three miserable years, for myself and family, a friend gave me an article on reflexology. I read it and thought that I should give it a try, I had nothing to lose. I found a qualified practitioner listed in a local telephone directory and went for several treatments. From the first treatment I found that my symptoms began to improve, my energy began to return, and I began to feel more relaxed and optimistic about life.

About the same time I was introduced to two other therapies: Reiki and the Bach Flower Remedies. Without any doubt these three therapies set me on the road to good health and inner well-being. Although I would not like to go through such an illness again, I do feel that I learned much from that time and the way my life has developed as a result of it has more than compensated for the distress and discomfort I experienced. I feel that I was redirected or put back on track or pointed in the right direction. Being ill gives us time to think and it often forces us to look at ourselves and our lives in a new light. It also helps us to understand what it is like to be ill and this gives us empathy and compassion for others who are suffering. These qualities are invaluable for therapists and healers.

I have gained great benefit from reflexology both personally and professionally. It is a wonderful, versatile, simple, and effective healing therapy. Anyone can practice it and everyone can benefit from it. The wish to write this book and share what I know of reflexology with others arose from the benefits I gained and those I have seen others derive from receiving reflexology, treating themselves and treating others.

Some of the most enjoyable, moving, and fulfilling reflexology treatments I have given have been at a hospice for cancer patients. If there was any doubt in my mind that reflexology was just a physical treatment without a spiritual aspect, then these were completely removed following these experiences. Many times I felt that the healing being received was on other subtle levels, from beyond the physical realm, especially on those patients without long to live. I also learned that the true meaning of healing is much more than just promoting good physical health. Simply letting go of your own worries, trusting in a positive outlook, directing your life toward benefiting others, and improving and understanding yourself is the path to inner peace and these qualities in turn are some of the basic ingredients of good health.

In the Footsteps of Buddha

While I was training to become a reflexologist our teacher told me of a Buddhist meditation center in the English Lake District (Cumbria) called Manjushri Center (www.manjushri.org.uk). I went to visit with a friend in order to learn a little more about meditation and simply to have a weekend out of the city where I lived. This was the beginning of a fascinating journey in to the heart of Tibetan Buddhism, which is continuing today. Much of what I have gained from studying Buddha's teachings and practicing meditation has helped me to gain a clearer and deeper understanding of how we can use reflexology to cure and prevent illness. I have found the Buddhist explanations on the cause and cure of disease, the nature of the mind, and the path to true freedom and happiness to be flawless, practical, and of great benefit to me as a reflexologist and simply as someone interested in being happy!

I thought that much of what I learned from Buddhism would be of great relevance and interest to other reflexologists and to those learning about this ancient healing art for the first time. There is no doubt that reflexology was being practiced in ancient India, where Buddha was born and grew up, as it forms part of the ancient Vedic healing arts. Before Buddha began his spiritual journey towards enlightenment he lived as a wealthy prince and heir to a vast kingdom and there, amongst other pleasures, he would more than likely have received reflexology himself in the royal palace. So it is quite nice in a way to bring these two things together again in a modern context.

There is no doubt that reflexology is a powerful, noninvasive, and effective healing technique. If this book is studied methodically and carefully it would be difficult to practice incorrectly and harm others. Although it does not take long to learn the basics in order to treat yourself, family, and friends it is important if you want to practice professionally to complete an appropriate course of study that leads to a recognized qualification. Then you should obtain the correct insurance before beginning your career as a reflexologist.

Reflexology is a very rewarding and fulfilling career, hobby, or pastime. It can easily become a lifelong interest and we can have much fun and gain great satisfaction in seeing the benefits we bring to friends, family, and other patients. I hope this book is interesting and helpful, and points you in the right direction if you are looking for one!

1

What Is Reflexology?

The *Oxford English Dictionary* describes reflexology as:

> *The practice of massaging points on the feet to relieve tension and treat illness.*

It describes a reflex as:

> *An involuntary or automatic movement in response to a stimulus.*

These are good, general descriptions, but they only scratch the surface of the true definition of the art and science of reflexology. Indeed, the definition of the word "reflex" is quite misleading. Reflexologists are not looking for a corresponding "movement," but rather another stimulus or reaction in the form of an increase, decrease, or rebalance of a particular physical, mental, or emotional function.

On one level, the aim of reflexology is simply and primarily to restore health to the body and mind as quickly and easily as possible, so that the patient needs no further treatment and can enjoy life again. Of course, it would be wonderful if that happened every time reflexology was used. However, we do not live in a perfect world, so the aim of reflexology has to be realistically adjusted to reflect what can be practically achieved with each individual patient.

Sometimes we may only achieve a reduction in the severity of the patient's symptoms, and this improvement might have to be maintained with regular treatments. However, we can regard such a treatment to be successful if the patient is happy with the improvements.

The patient's attitude to his or her condition is of paramount importance. This is where reflexology can have the most profound effects. Encouraging positive mental and emotional qualities throughout the treatment, listening, and sometimes talking to the patients are some of the best ways reflexologists can help them. A positive mind is a wonderful byproduct of receiving reflexology and one of the most important factors in the healing process. We can even verify the power of a positive mind on one's health through the results of scientific research. It's official: Being happy is good for you!

In fact, restoring a good mental attitude should be a reflexologist's number one priority. We will look at the reasons for this later, but for now we can definitely say that a happy mind is a very useful thing. There are many people in this world who have to deal with severe suffering of one form or another, yet many do so with a happy mind, a contented mind, a mind that wishes no more than that very happiness. Are such people healthy? Do they need healing?

What relevance does this have to a definition or understanding of reflexology? If we are embarking on a journey toward an understanding of the "way of healing," then, from the start, we need to develop some wisdom to temper and shape the power of our compassionate wish to help others. Wisdom is essential. You can be the most technically accomplished and compassionate healer, but without a little wisdom, many of your actions can be misguided and your time and effort wasted. Strange as it may seem, good health is not the "be all and end all" of the healer's ambition. Again, we will examine this later when we look at the cause and cure of disease and the nature of the mind (chapter 8).

How Reflexology Works

It really is impossible to say when reflexology was first used. The oldest known documentation of reflexology is depicted on the wall of a tomb of an Egyptian physician called Ankmahor, located in Saqqara, Egypt. It dates back to around 2330–2500 B.C. and shows two men working on the feet of two other men. In the inscription the patient says, "Do not hurt me," and the therapist replies, "I shall act so you praise me." (See appendix 1 for more on the history of reflexology.)

If we regard foot massage as a simple type of reflexology, then we can say that reflexology is as old as the human race—perhaps older. Many types of monkeys, including those most closely related to humans, perform a primitive type of foot massage. Obviously, they do not consciously realize that they are stimulating the body's healing powers. It is simply instinctive and it feels good. Many people like to have their feet massaged. It is relaxing, enjoyable, and relieves stress in many ways. But there is a definite difference between foot massage and reflexology, although both benefit the body and mind for the same reasons.

There are two main schools of thought as to how reflexology actually works. Unfortunately, at present, neither can be clinically proven to be correct. However, that does not seem to change the fact that reflexology works.

The first theory that many of the original reflexologists preferred, including Eunice Ingham, who is considered the mother of modern reflexology, was that the foot is linked to various parts of the body by a countless number of nerve endings. There are an unusually large number of nerve endings in the feet, and that is why many people find their feet particularly sensitive to physical stimulation like tickling. It was and still is thought that the various nerve endings correspond to "zones" of the body, called zone theory. Dr. William Fitzgerald discovered that the body could be divided into ten vertical zones, running from head to toe and corresponding to the ten fingers and ten toes. (See Figure 1.) Pressure applied on certain fingers would have

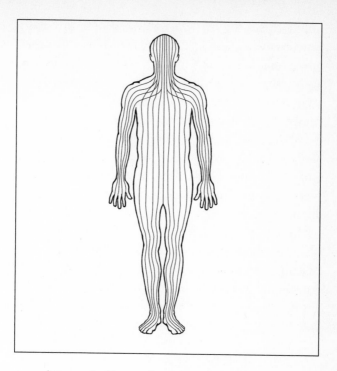

Figure 1: *Illustration of the zones of the body based on zone theory*

an effect on parts of the body contained within the corresponding zones.

It was also thought that the nerve endings corresponded to the map of the human anatomy. In fact, if we look at the soles of our feet together, they appear to form the general shape of the human body: the big toes relate to the head and neck of the torso; the base of the little toes are the left and right shoulders; and each instep is the left and right side of the spine.

To some extent, this theory is also true, but there is no definite evidence that makes it a conclusive, accurate, and definitive theory. In fact, the number and complexity of nerve endings in the feet make it almost impossible to clearly identify which areas of the feet affect which parts of the body. Because the nervous system is so extensive and covers the whole body, creating pleasure or pain in just one small area has a dramatic effect on the whole.

Despite this lack of scientific conclusions, there is plenty of evidence from case studies and anecdotes that practicing reflexology rather than simple foot massage has such a beneficial effect on health that we have to admit that massaging and stimulating the feet in a specific way has a direct and positive effect on the body and mind.

Many healers nowadays explain reflexology through their knowledge of Chinese medicine. This stipulates that there are within the body a number of invisible energy pathways, or meridians, that carry life force energy, or chi/ki. It is said that when these pathways become blocked, perhaps due to stress, then illness can result. Sometimes acupuncture or acupressure is used to release these blockages and stimulate a free flow of healthy life force energy. As most of the major energy pathways end or begin in the feet, so naturally reflexology will stimulate them in some way. However, even a full reflexology treatment would not stimulate or treat all of the meridians as they do not all end in the feet, and there are many minor or tributary pathways as well as the main ones. This is why acupuncture and acupressure are performed all over the body. (Acupuncture is many thousands of years old, so if it were most effective by treating only the feet, one would think this would have been noticed by now.)

Some New Ideas

We really have to look for some new clues and simple ideas as to why reflexology works as well as acupuncture and other similar therapies. One possible explanation that takes something from both the nerve ending theory, or zone theory, and the life force meridian theory is as follows.

We know from many of the Eastern philosophies and systems of natural medicine that the nervous system is the link between the mind and body. We also know that the subtle internal energies, or "winds" as they are known in Buddhist philosophy, govern our mental and physical health. When we are carrying and naturally generating strong, clear, and well-balanced subtle internal winds, then our physical and mental health is good. To understand these ideas, it will be helpful to gain a basic understanding of what life force energy is and why it is so important and vital to life.

We could say that life force energy is the subtle foundation of all life, a sort of cosmic soup that supports, nourishes, and sustains the cycle of birth, life, and death of all forms of life.

Modern physics tells us that all matter is made up of differing frequencies of energy. Solid objects are made up of energy vibrating at a very low or slow frequency. Less solid objects like water, air, and life force energy are vibrating incredibly fast. We also know that within the molecules and atoms of matter there is proportionately more space than between the planets in the universe, so all is not as it seems.

Many of the Eastern philosophies like Buddhism and Vedic science understand the concept of energy much better than we do. They also incorporate this knowledge into their religions in a way that explains the mystical and spiritual experiences that many devoted practitioners have. In these societies, science, religion, and art are not separated but are seen simply as branches of the same tree of life. One aspect of the Eastern understanding of God is as a universal life force energy; that is, the one true source of all life. All the energy that breathes life into plants, trees, animals, humans, planets, stars, and universes comes from this one source. It is this source of life that we need to make contact with if we want to maintain or recreate good physical, mental, and spiritual health.

When we are in touch with this energy through prayer, meditation, taking a walk in the countryside, or receiving healing, we feel less "separate" and increasingly "whole" within ourselves and within the "whole" of creation. We experience a sense of unity. We become more aware of our place or role in the great scheme of things, and at the same time we feel supported, safe, open, and confident in our abilities to be all that we are, without doubt or apology. We can say that these spiritual or personal experiences are the "essence" of healing, and are a pleasant byproduct of many complimentary therapies.

There are two main types of life force energy: internal and external. Internal life force energy is the subtle energy that exists within the body and mind of all living beings. External life force energy exists within plants, flowers, trees, rocks, minerals, and crystals. This energy is often harnessed for healing purposes as in the Bach Flower Remedies, crystal healing, and homeopathic and herbal remedies. Even just a walk in the woods or by the sea can have a calming and healing effect on us. There is so much pure external life force energy available in these places that it "lifts" our own internal energies, and this has a corresponding effect on our body and mind. Conversely, if we spend too much time in urban areas or stressful environments where these natural energies are restricted, this may adversely affect our health, especially if we are unable to transform or rise above these situations. As mentioned before, internal life force energy runs through subtle channels or meridians in the human body, and when these are blocked or unbalanced, due to stress for example, illness can result. Most complementary therapies seek to help the body and mind rebalance and cleanse these internal energies, thereby promoting health and wellbeing, and this is also the way reflexology works as a healing technique.

Reflexology can have a profound effect on our health and well-being by rebalancing, cleansing, and renewing our internal energy system. When internal life force energy is blocked, sluggish, or unbalanced, regular reflexology treatments have the effect of naturally and effortlessly dissolving and raising the quality of that energy to the healthiest level that our body, mind, and environment will allow. A reflexology treatment also has the effect of opening our energy system to again receive a well-balanced flow of universal life force energy that is often cut off or restricted by illness. Perhaps more accurately we can say that being cut off from this life force is the cause of much illness.

So a big part of the healing process is to establish why the patient became distant from his or her natural relationship with the universal life force, and how they can work to maintain a healthy relationship with it in the future. For some this may involve a personal spiritual revolution, by rediscovering his or her own religion or a new religion, or perhaps looking into such practices as meditation, yoga, or Tai Chi. We do not have to become religious to develop this special inner relationship with life. Babies are not necessarily religious, but they definitely carry a special pure energy that comes from somewhere special. It is interesting to note that many well-known and respected spiritual teachers, healers, and saints carry a similar energy.

Conscious Energy

When internal and external life force energy are in harmony, possess the same level of purity, exist on the same wavelength/frequency, and are within the same realm of existence, they are very similar energies. The only difference is that internal life force energy has consciousness or "mind" and cannot exist separately from it. Due to the close relationship between consciousness and internal life force energy, it is easy to believe that the sense of closeness or companionship we feel toward trees, crystals, the Earth, or other sources of external life force energy is because they possess a personal character or mind. External life force energy, like that within trees, crystals, and the Earth, does not possess consciousness or mind. However, this does not make them any less special or sacred "living" objects.

So our internal energies and our mind are inseparable. They exist almost as one and have a very intimate, dependent relationship. In fact, although we do not generally notice it, our thoughts and feelings "ride" on our internal energies. If we carry positive internal life force energy of a good quality, it is easier for us to develop positive states of mind, and we generally attract positive life experiences and deal with problems more easily. Likewise, if we consciously try to develop positive states of mind like confidence, kindness, and wisdom, this will raise the quality of our internal energies and, in turn, improve our health and many other aspects of our lives.

Linking the Ancient and Modern

Coming back to the link between the nervous system, the mind, and our internal energies, we can say that the practice of reflexology stimulates or relaxes the nervous system. This, in turn, affects the mind and our internal energy system at the same time, as they are inseparable. As will be explained in more detail later, if we possess the potential to get well, then simply by treating, stimulating, relaxing, or "massaging" the mind and internal energy system through the nervous system, we will naturally move toward good health. Our bodies tend to do this anyway given the right conditions. What we are doing in reflexology and other therapies is simply encouraging this process and creating the inner peace, "space," and other conditions conducive to healing.

It is truly amazing to see the positive changes in physical and mental health that arise just from massaging the feet. Much of this is simply due to the deep physical and mental relaxation created during a reflexology treatment, as this is one of the major conditions required for us to regain our own inner healing abilities. There are many other obvious conditions like good diet, regular exercise, social and environmental circumstances, mental attitude, etc. However, there are times when good health is not so easily restored or maintained; then we need to look for deeper solutions. (These will be examined later in chapter 8 on the cause and cure of disease.)

Generally speaking, we can see that with good motivation, reflexology can greatly assist us in improving our own quality of life and that of others, helping us become more whole and healthy beings on all levels. This, in turn, naturally benefits those around us and the friends and relatives of those we treat. When we help a patient, we are indirectly helping all those people that our patient has a close connection or relationship with. What a special opportunity to benefit others.

2

Locating the Reflexes

Gaining an accurate understanding of how the human anatomy is reflected in the foot reflexes is the key to good reflexology. The following illustrations and text explain in detail the major foot reflexes and how they relate to the different systems and parts of the body.

It will seem at first as though there is a lot of information to digest. The major reflexes for the head, spine, lungs, and intestines are fairly easy to locate and memorize. However, you do not need to memorize all of this information before being able to practice successful reflexology. You can refer back to these illustrations as you continue learning the techniques. Then as you become more accomplished and confident, you can deepen your knowledge by trying to memorize where the more intricate reflexes are located.

Some bodily functions or organs are so basic that they need no explanation, whereas others are so complex that a full description would be impossible in a book of this nature. It is recommended that the reader use a comprehensive guide to anatomy and physiology to gain a detailed knowledge. Such knowledge is essential if you wish to practice professionally, and it will form a key part of any practitioner's course. However, if you are happy to practice on friends and family, the simple explanations that follow are more than adequate.

Beginning with the toes, which represent the head and neck area, we will examine the major anatomical parts influenced by these foot reflexes. Then working toward the heels and ankles we will look at the area between the shoulders and diaphragm, which corresponds to the ball of the foot. We will move to the abdominal area, which corresponds to the reflexes between the ball of the foot and the heel, and then to the pelvic area, which reflects the heel itself. Next the inner aspect of the foot relating to the spine is explained, then the outer aspect relating to the arms, hips, legs, etc., and finally, the top of the foot for the additional chest and circulation reflexes.

Although we are moving systematically down the foot from toe to heel, many of the reflexes relating to different parts or systems overlap. An explanation of a particular system, like the nervous, lymphatic, or pulmonary system, is given in the most appropriate place possible. Obvious anatomical explanations for things like teeth, eyes, or arms are not given.

Toes/Head and Neck Area

Endocrine System

The endocrine system is made up of various glands that secrete different types of hormones directly into the bloodstream. The main endocrine glands are the pituitary, thyroid, parathyroid, adrenal, ovary and testes, placenta, and part of the pancreas. Through hormones they control the chemical composition, function, and stasis or balance of the body. Hormones are very potent chemical substances that, once produced, are carried around the body to different organs or tissues, which recognize or respond to them, and subsequently alter their function or structure according to the type of hormone present. Every organ and tissue in the body is controlled by very complex chemical actions and reactions. Chemically, the body is in a constant state of flux or inner motion, and the endocrine system serves to control and balance all this inner activity.

(Refer to Figure 2, page 18.)

Pituitary: (Reflex #7) This is sometimes referred to as the master endocrine gland. It is about the size of a pea and is attached to the hypothalamus at the base of the skull. It secretes various important hormones.

Hypothalamus: (Reflex #11) This controls body temperature, hunger, water balance, and sexual function. It is also the center of cooperation or communication between the hormone and autonomic nervous system.

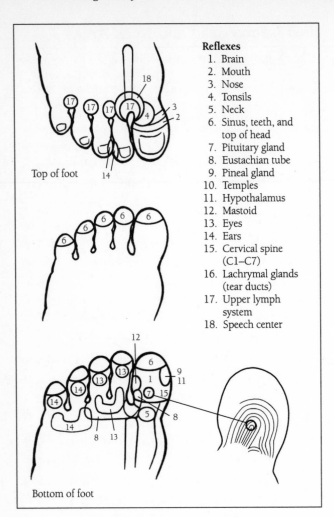

Reflexes
1. Brain
2. Mouth
3. Nose
4. Tonsils
5. Neck
6. Sinus, teeth, and top of head
7. Pituitary gland
8. Eustachian tube
9. Pineal gland
10. Temples
11. Hypothalamus
12. Mastoid
13. Eyes
14. Ears
15. Cervical spine (C1–C7)
16. Lachrymal glands (tear ducts)
17. Upper lymph system
18. Speech center

Top of foot

Bottom of foot

Figure 2: *Reflexes on the toes relating to the head and neck area*

Head Reflexes

Ears and inner ear: (Reflex #14) The inner ear or "labyrinth" is a system of cavities and ducts that form the organs of hearing and balance, including the Eustachian tube (Reflex #8), which connects the middle ear to the pharynx.

Tonsils: (Reflex #4) These are small masses of lymphatic tissue that help to prevent infections.

Other Areas

Pineal gland: (Reflex #9) This is a pea-sized area of nerve tissue attached to the third ventricle of the brain. It is a gland that produces the hormone melatonin (a derivative of seratonin, which can be found throughout the body), which helps to regulate the sleep cycle (along with seratonin).

Mastoid: (Reflex #12) This refers to two things: mastoid process—a nipple-shaped protrusion on the temporal bone that extends downward and forward behind the ear canal; mastoid antrum—an air-filled channel connecting the mastoid process to the cavity of the middle ear.

Cervical spine: (Reflex #15) These are the seven bones making up the neck region of the spinal column. (See also pages 31–34.)

Lachrymal glands or tear ducts: (Reflex #16) (See also pages 36–37.)

Upper lymphatic system: (Reflex #17) This is the network of vessels (in the upper part of the body, especially around the armpits, neck, and central chest area) that convey lymph (electrolytes, water, proteins, etc.) from the tissue fluids to the bloodstream. It makes up a major part of the immune system. (See also pages 36–37.)

Speech center: (Reflex #18) This is the part of the brain that controls speech. (See also pages 36–37.)

Ball of the Foot/Thoracic Region

Respiratory and Circulatory Systems

Circulation causes the blood to flow through the body over 1,000 times a day. It provides all the major organs with what they need to function effectively, enables the immune system to operate, and continually removes and expels toxins.

Blood is vitally oxygenated in the lungs and travels from the left side of the heart to all parts of the body, constantly regenerating and feeding the vital organs on the way back to the heart. The blood is cleaned and toxins are removed along the way, and the process begins again. Red blood cells carry oxygen around the body, and white blood cells fight disease and infection, cleaning the blood and body of impurities. The production of white blood cells is increased during times of illness and/or infection.

The respiratory and cardiac systems are closely related, almost like two ends of a seesaw. When one is

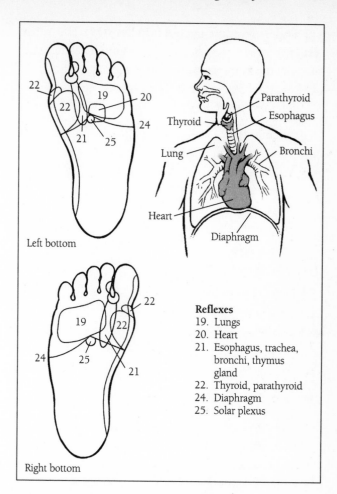

Reflexes
19. Lungs
20. Heart
21. Esophagus, trachea, bronchi, thymus gland
22. Thyroid, parathyroid
24. Diaphragm
25. Solar plexus

Figure 3: *Reflexes on the ball of the foot relating to the thoracic region*

put under pressure by physical exertion, the other responds, and vice versa, until they find a balance that supplies the body with the amount of oxygen and rate of blood flow that it needs to continue.

(Refer to Figure 3, page 21.)

Bronchial tree: (Reflex #21) A branching system of tubes from the base connection with the trachea to the tips of the bronchi and bronchioles, the smallest branches, which open into the alveoli. There the gas exchange takes place with the blood capillaries surrounding them: oxygen going into the blood, and waste gases being released for expulsion through exhalation.

Diaphragm: (Reflex #24) A thin, dome-shaped muscle that separates the thoracic and abdominal cavities, playing a major role in respiration by stretching and expanding the lungs downward upon inhalation.

Other Reflexes

Thymus gland: (Reflex #21) This gland is part of the immune system. Its main function is during infancy and before puberty. It controls the growth and development of a major part of the immune system.

Thyroid and parathyroid: (Reflex #22) These are part of the endocrine system. The two main lobes of the thyroid gland mainly regulate the metabolic rate of the body including mental and physical development. Excessive amounts of or a lack of thyroid hormones leads to ill-health. Behind or slightly within the thyroid are the parathyroid glands. These produce the hormones that control the distribution of calcium and phosphate in the body.

Solar plexus: (Reflex #25) Part of the nervous system, it is a complex and densely packed area of nerves forming part of the autonomic system located high in the back of the abdomen. It is a sensitive and important reflex for helping the whole body and mind relax.

Arch of the Foot/Abdominal Area

Digestive System

The digestive system transforms food and drink into simple, nutritional forms that various bodily functions require to sustain them. Ingestion is the first part of the process, which ends with the secretion of waste. In between there is a complex process of breaking down the food and drink and absorbing what is required, ready for use.

(Refer to Figure 4, page 24. The dotted lines simply indicate how the foot can be mentally split into sections to help you identify the reflex areas.)

Esophagus/cardiac sphincter: (Reflex #21, Figure 3, page 21.) The esophagus leads from the back of the mouth to the stomach, and is lined with a mucous membrane that helps to lubricate the passage of food into the stomach. The cardiac

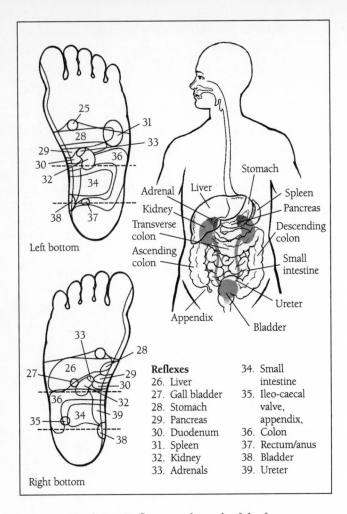

Left bottom

Right bottom

Stomach
Adrenal / Liver
Spleen
Kidney
Pancreas
Transverse colon
Descending colon
Ascending colon
Small intestine
Ureter
Appendix
Bladder

Reflexes
26. Liver
27. Gall bladder
28. Stomach
29. Pancreas
30. Duodenum
31. Spleen
32. Kidney
33. Adrenals

34. Small intestine
35. Ileo-caecal valve, appendix,
36. Colon
37. Rectum/anus
38. Bladder
39. Ureter

Figure 4: *Reflexes on the arch of the foot relating to the abdominal area*

sphincter is a ring of muscle that controls entry into the stomach.

Stomach/pyloric sphincter: (Reflex #28) The stomach lies mainly to the left side of the body and forms a large, muscular sack, which transforms food by chemically and mechanically blending and homogenizing it into a creamy substance known as chime. The pyloric sphincter is located at the exit of the stomach and is similar to the cardiac sphincter. Between them they control the amount of food entering and leaving the stomach.

Liver: (Reflex #26) Situated on the upper right of the abdomen, the liver produces bile for digestion, which drains into the gall bladder before being released into the duodenum. The liver also regulates blood sugar, removes excess amino acids, and stores and metabolizes fats, proteins, and carbohydrates. It also acts to detoxify the body and produces various other important chemicals.

Gall bladder: (Reflex #27) Located under the right side of the liver, the gall bladder stores bile for use in digestion.

Pancreas: (Reflex #29) Found behind the stomach, it forms and releases pancreatic juices into the duodenum through the pancreatic duct. Within the pancreas is a group of cells known as the Islet of Langerhans, which secrete insulin and glucagon hormones into the bloodstream.

Small intestine: (Reflex #34) The first part of the small intestine is the duodenum. It stretches from the stomach to the jejunum, the second part of the system. It receives bile and pancreatic juices to help the digestion process. The jejunum leads to the ileum, the lowest of the three parts of the small intestine. It ends in the ileo-caecal valve, which controls entry into the large intestine and prevents backflow into the ileum.

Appendix: (Reflex #25) This is a short tube, with no obvious important purpose, attached to the digestive system, close to the junction of the small and large intestine. There is some secretion into the large intestine, which helps to lubricate digestion, and it also contains lymphatic material for the immune system.

Large intestine (Reflex #36) About five feet in length, it surrounds the small intestine by ascending, transversing, and descending on the left side of the body. The junctions between these three parts are called the hepatic flexure, splenic flexure, and sigmoid flexure, respectively. The sigmoid flexure leads into the rectum and then the anus. All along the route, digested food takes the necessary nutrients, vitamins, minerals, and fats that are absorbed through the walls of the small and large intestines. Those nutrients, like fats that require more time to digest, are broken down and absorbed into the body in the large intestine. Those that can be assimilated more quickly are dealt with earlier on in the process in the small intestine, the stomach, and even in the esophagus.

Colon: (Reflex #36) This is the main part of the large intestine composing four parts: the ascending, transverse, descending, and the sigmoid colon. The colon absorbs large amounts of water and electrolytes from undigested food.

Other Reflexes

Adrenals: (Reflex #33) Adrenals are part of the endocrine system. Covering the upper part of each kidney, these glands produce adrenaline and corticosteroid hormones. Adrenaline affects the muscles, circulation, and sugar levels within the body. Corticosteroid is a type of steroid.

Main Parts of the Urinary System

Kidneys: (Reflex #32) The kidneys cleanse the blood of soluble impurities and toxins, principally urea, and regulate water and mineral balance. The nephrons within the kidney filter the blood then reabsorb water and selected substances back into the blood.

Ureter: (Reflex #39) This muscular tube connects the kidneys with the bladder and transmits urine.

Bladder: (Reflex #38) It temporarily holds/stores urine for expulsion.

Heel/Pelvic Area

(Refer to Figure 5.)

Sciatic and pelvic area: (Reflex #41) The sciatic nerve is the main nerve of the leg. It is the largest nerve in the body and runs from the end of the spine down behind the thigh.

Ankle/Reproductive Organs

(Refer to Figure 6, page 30.)

Ovaries: (Reflex #42) The female reproductive organs containing follicles that produce ova and steroid hormones in regular cycles.

Testes: (Reflex #42) The male reproductive glands producing spermatozoa and the male hormone testosterone.

Uterus: (Reflex #43) Located in the central pelvic cavity in females, it functions to nourish and protect the fetus during pregnancy.

Prostate: (Reflex #43) Found at the base of the bladder in males. Opening into the urethra, it produces fluid to carry and protect sperm.

Fallopian tubes: (Reflex #44) These connect the ovaries with the uterus and transport the ova from the ovaries to the uterus during ovulation.

Urethra: (Reflex #47) The tube that expels urine from the bladder, ending at the tip of the penis in men, and just within the vulva in women.

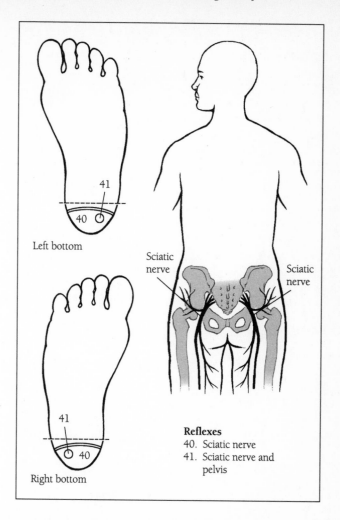

Figure 5: *Reflexes in the heels relating to the pelvic area*

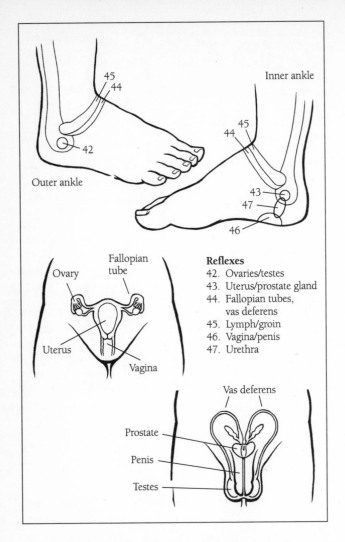

Figure 6: *Reflexes on the ankles relating to the reproductive organs*

Vas deferens: (Reflex #44) These carry semen from the prostate to the urethra.

Inner Foot/Spine

The spine consists of thirty-three vertebrae and is divided into five sections. It is the central support of the body and a main constituent in the nervous and skeletal system.

Looking at Figure 7, page 32, and Figure 8, page 33, there are a lot of reflexes relating to the inner foot/spine. Again, you do not need to treat just a few reflexes at one time, but always try to do a whole treatment. Locating the reflexes comes from studying the diagrams, looking and treating lots of different types of feet, intuition (which comes with experience), and comparing notes with other reflexologists. A beginner could pretend that the reflex is larger than it is and treat this larger area so as to be sure that the reflex is covered properly. You don't have to pinpoint accurately at the start. Just covering the whole foot using the massage techniques explained will be almost as effective.

Nervous System

The nervous system is a vast network of cells specifically designed to transmit nerve impulses or "information" to and from all areas of the body in order to bring about, monitor, and control all bodily activities, from the smallest adjustments at the microscopic level to the functions of all the major organs. It is the body's information highway.

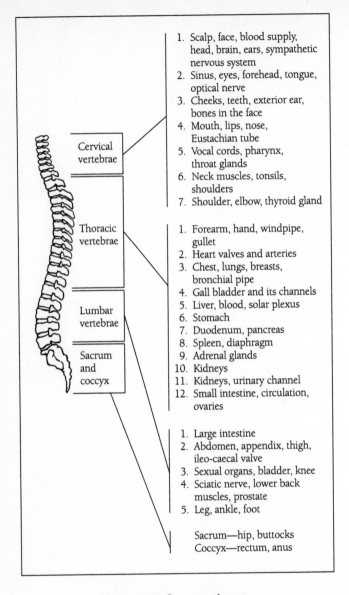

Cervical vertebrae
1. Scalp, face, blood supply, head, brain, ears, sympathetic nervous system
2. Sinus, eyes, forehead, tongue, optical nerve
3. Cheeks, teeth, exterior ear, bones in the face
4. Mouth, lips, nose, Eustachian tube
5. Vocal cords, pharynx, throat glands
6. Neck muscles, tonsils, shoulders
7. Shoulder, elbow, thyroid gland

Thoracic vertebrae
1. Forearm, hand, windpipe, gullet
2. Heart valves and arteries
3. Chest, lungs, breasts, bronchial pipe
4. Gall bladder and its channels
5. Liver, blood, solar plexus
6. Stomach
7. Duodenum, pancreas
8. Spleen, diaphragm
9. Adrenal glands
10. Kidneys
11. Kidneys, urinary channel
12. Small intestine, circulation, ovaries

Lumbar vertebrae
1. Large intestine
2. Abdomen, appendix, thigh, ileo-caecal valve
3. Sexual organs, bladder, knee
4. Sciatic nerve, lower back muscles, prostate
5. Leg, ankle, foot

Sacrum and coccyx
Sacrum—hip, buttocks
Coccyx—rectum, anus

Figure 7: Reflexes on the spine

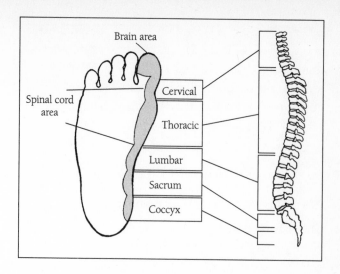

Figure 8: *How the spine reflexes
relate to the inner foot*

The nervous system has three main parts: the central nervous system, the peripheral nervous system, and the autonomic nervous system. The central nervous system is responsible for the integration of all nerve activities, like a central mainframe computer. Its main components are the brain and spinal cord within the spinal column. The peripheral nervous system is all the other parts of the nervous system, other than the central nervous system, and this includes the cranial and spinal nerves. The autonomic nervous system is part of the peripheral system. It controls those parts of the body that the conscious mind has no regular or direct control over those parts of the body that need no conscious effort to work: the beating of the heart; sweating;

intestinal movements; and the growth, development, and aging of the body. The autonomic system is again divided into two parts: the sympathetic nervous system and the parasympathetic system. It is through the autonomic nervous system that many people believe reflexology works.

Outer Foot/Outer Body

Muscular and Skeletal System

The skeletal system gives the body form, a strong and rigid framework allowing mobility, and serves to protect and support vital organs. The main quality of muscle fiber is that it has the ability to contract, producing movement of force.

(Refer to Figure 9.)

Ribs, sternum, clavicle, and scapular: The sternum is better known as the chest bone, and the clavicles and scapular are known as the collar bone and shoulder blade, respectively.

Hands: Running from the wrist to the fingers, the main bones are the carpals, metacarpals, and phalanges.

Feet: Running from the ankle to the toes, the main bones are the tarsals, metatarsals, and phalanges.

Arms: This includes the upper arm bone, or humerus, and the lower arm bones: radius (largest) and ulna.

Legs: Includes the thigh bone, or femur, and the lower leg bones: tibia (largest) and fibula.

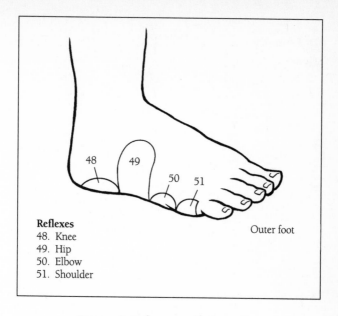

Reflexes
48. Knee
49. Hip
50. Elbow
51. Shoulder

Outer foot

*Figure 9: Reflexes on the outer foot
relating to the outer body*

Top of the Foot/Lymphatic System

Lymphatic System

Forming a major part of the body's immune system, the lymphatic system is made up of a network of lymph nodes and channels. Lymph—which consists of proteins, electrolytes, and water—is carried from tissue fluids to the bloodstream. The lymphatic vessels or channels lead to two large channels: the right lymphatic duct and the thoracic duct, which return the lymph to the bloodstream. This system needs the movement of

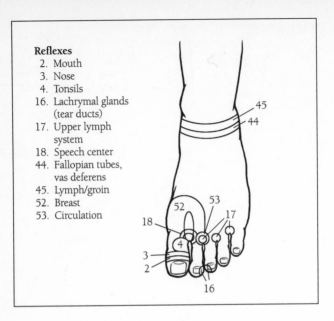

Reflexes
2. Mouth
3. Nose
4. Tonsils
16. Lachrymal glands
(tear ducts)
17. Upper lymph
system
18. Speech center
44. Fallopian tubes,
vas deferens
45. Lymph/groin
52. Breast
53. Circulation

Figure 10: *Reflexes on the top of the foot
relating to the lymphatic system*

the body, as well as respiration and gravity, to work most effectively. It works to fight disease and infection and removes everyday toxins from the body.

(Refer to Figure 10.)

Upper lymphatics: (Reflex #17) These are mainly located in the head, neck, armpits, and central chest area. (See also Figure 2, page 18.)

Lower lymphatics: (Reflex #45) These are mainly located around the solar plexus/stomach area, spleen, groin, and behind the knees. (See also Figure 6, page 30.)

Other Areas

Lachrymal glands: (See also pages 18–20.)

Speech center: (See also pages 18–20.)

Fallopian tube/vas deferens: (See also pages 28–30.)

3

Basic Techniques

The basic techniques that are used during a reflexology treatment cannot be learned quickly. It really takes years to master them until they become second nature. You can best notice the difference by receiving a treatment from a newly qualified reflexologist and someone who has been practicing for many years.

However, reflexology is such an effective and powerful form of therapy that even in the hands of the inexperienced remarkable and lasting healing can take place in just a short time. You should not be afraid to expect success and good results right from the beginning. If you take your time and do not rush to learn all there is to know, even your very first treatment will be effective.

It's important to take time to learn and practice the basics. If you have a friend or partner who is willing to be the patient, you should take advantage of that as often as possible and practice all the techniques whenever you can.

Giving a reflexology treatment will involve using your hands to apply pressure and different types of massage to the feet in specific ways. The techniques are simple but require practice and patience to perfect them.

Initially you may feel more comfortable practicing the basic techniques on your own hands or feet. You will immediately gain experience on how the techniques might feel to a patient. You will also learn how much pressure to apply, which is important for the patient's comfort and saves the therapist's muscles from strain.

Treating the feet and performing the different types of hand movements do not require great strength. The best reflexologists are not the strongest, so don't think that bulging muscles and strenuous massage are required. But the techniques will make your fingers, hands, and arms stronger. Initially, your shoulders may feel some strain before they become stronger, so it is helpful to pace yourself and not take on too much, perhaps just a few treatments per week as a start. Eventually you may be able to do several per day, depending on your own strength, although quality is always better than quantity.

When you are treating others, be prepared to adapt to their needs. Some feet are very sensitive, and if the patient is ill and has never had reflexology before, the first few treatments may need to be very light. Some parts of the feet may be much more sensitive than others, so again, the first treatment should be a gentle exploration, noting those areas that need a lighter touch. This also helps to recognize progress in the treatment: When sensitive areas become less painful, this is a good sign that the corresponding physical anatomy is reacting well to the treatment.

Light Touch or Deep Massage?

Reflexologists generally use a combination of light touch and deep massage. Some reflexologists never use a deep massage technique, because they feel it is ineffective and can, if used without thought, cause pain and discomfort to the patient. In some Chinese forms of reflexology, deep massage is the only technique used along with even more brutal techniques that use short sticks to press deep into the sole of the foot. There is no doubt that such treatments can be painful, and the cries and shouts of patients can often be heard outside the clinic! However, there is also no doubt that such treatments are very effective and have been for thousands of years.

Modern Western reflexology is not like this. Although deep massage can be applied using techniques like the knuckle press, you should only use them when you have gained enough experience. You should never use deep massage if the patient experiences pain, although some discomfort is acceptable if the patient is genuinely accepting of this. Once you learn when to apply more pressure, these deep massage techniques can be very effective when used sparingly. Again, never use deep massage in the first or second treatment of a new client unless you are sure it is wise to do so!

You can cover an area two or three times until you are satisfied it has be properly stimulated, although overstimulation of reflexes is to be avoided, especially in the very ill, children, pregnant women, particularly sensitive people, and those patients coming for their first or second treatment.

Some reflexologists always use a very light touch, and this is also an effective technique. It certainly allows the patient to relax and seems to induce a subtle yet deep state of healing, particularly helpful for patients with mental and emotional problems.

As an individual therapist, you need to practice and find your own way of doing things. The way that naturally feels right to you is usually the best and most effective. There is no reason not to use a different technique with different types of patients according to their needs and your experience and confidence.

The following are the basic reflexology techniques. These are the most important techniques to learn and are used often throughout a treatment. They are not difficult to master with a little practice, and the best place to practice at first is simply on your own hands or feet. This enables you to feel how much pressure you are applying.

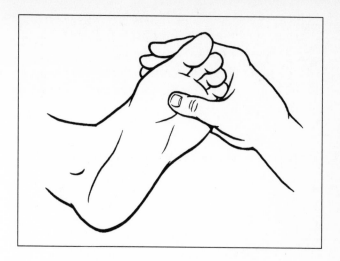

Figure 11: *Basic foot support hold*

Supporting Foot Hold

This basic support hold is used often throughout a treatment. While one hand is working a particular set of reflexes, the other hand is always used to support the foot. The idea is to prevent the foot from moving around too much, so a firm but gentle grip is needed.

For this basic foot hold, firmly but gently grab the top of the patient's foot, with your fingers on top of the toes and your thumb on the ball of the foot. (See Figure 11.) For best results, when working on reflexes on the inside of the patient's right foot, use your right hand as the support. When working on the outside of the foot, use your left hand as the support. This pattern is then reversed to work on the left foot.

Make sure not to bend the toes forward, and do not stretch the foot too far in any direction. Remember, the patient's comfort is always paramount.

Other support grips are used, for example, cupping the back of the heel. This hold and others are shown in the full treatment sequence in chapter 5.

Finger or Thumb Walking Technique

This massage technique is one of the most basic and often-used throughout a treatment. Again, the best way to practice the motion and level of pressure is on your own hand. Support the back of one hand with the fingers of the other hand. Gently press the thumb into the palm. (See Figure 12.) Release the pressure slowly while at the same time sliding the thumb forward slightly. Then apply gentle pressure again. Release, move forward, apply pressure, etc. This is called "thumb walking."

The main point is that there should be no gaps or spaces between the pressure points so that not even the smallest area of skin is missed. The action should be repeated constantly while trying to move in a straight line across the palm. The whole movement is a sort of rhythmic nibbling action.

If you are right-handed, you will probably find it easier to use your right thumb, but with practice you will be able to use both thumbs as easily. This is important as both hands are needed to be used equally during a full treatment.

This same nibbling or walking massage action is used with the fingers. This is usually performed with the

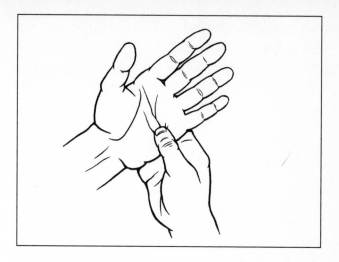

Figure 12: Thumb walking technique
practiced on the hand

index finger alone or the index and second finger
together.

Some reflexologists like to combine the finger and
thumb walking movements with a small rotating
motion, so that as pressure is applied, you move the
thumb in a tiny circular motion, usually clockwise. This
is repeated with every move forward. You might like
this technique and find it simple to use and very effective. However, if you find it difficult, just use the normal
technique to begin with; you can always come back to
this later. During a treatment, you could use both techniques when you feel it is right. Getting feedback from
the patient is also a helpful indicator.

Finger and Thumb Massage

This technique is a simple rubbing or massaging action. Figure 13 shows the index finger being used to massage the top and side of a toe. The thumb helps to support the toe. The other hand is employed in the basic support hold. (See Figure 11, page 43.) Simply rub the index finger back and forth in the area to be massaged. Again, some reflexologists use an additional circular motion, so you can try this if it feels right. You can also practice this technique on your fingers.

The two-finger massage technique is shown in Figure 14. Here the index and second fingers are being used together to massage the top of the foot (which is the reflex for the pelvic area, reproductive organs, and lymphatic system). The technique used is similar to the finger or thumb walking (see pages 44–45), although a circular motion is also employed as the fingers "nibble" along. Some reflexologists remove the nibble action here and simply use the circular massage action.

Pressure Technique and Knuckle Press/Massage

There are two types of massage used here. The first involves gently pinching and holding the heel with the thumb and index finger—the pressure technique. (See Figure 15, page 48.) This hold also supports the foot. The second type uses one or two knuckles to knead the area. (See Figure 15, page 48.) A little more pressure is usually applied to the heel area as it is usually covered by toughened skin, and the reflexes are located

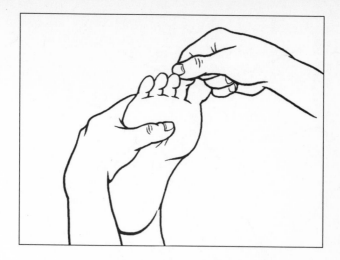

Figure 13: *Finger massage technique*

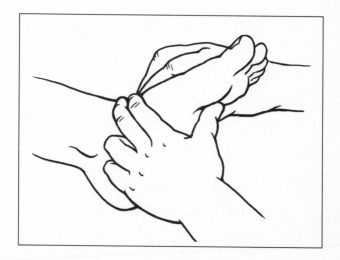

Figure 14: *Two-finger massage technique*

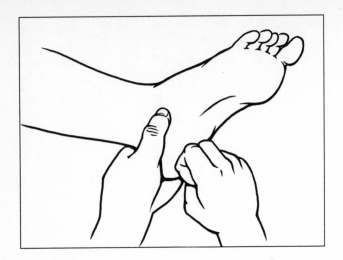

Figure 15: *Knuckle press technique (kneading)*

further below the surface. The knuckle can be pressed in and dragged down, or pressed in and gently rotated, moving slightly, and pressed and rotated again, and so on. Alternatively, a kneading action can be used, as though you were kneading bread. You can work from left to right or top to bottom as long as the whole heel area is covered.

Pressure Point Hold (Knuckle or Thumb)

Some reflexologists find that certain areas of the feet respond well to a simple pressure hold. A need for this might be indicated by skin that seems limp, puffy, or lacking "energy." Find the center of this area and press with a finger or thumb. The pressure should be no more than is comfortable for the patient, and should last between five to ten seconds, occasionally longer, and can be repeated two or three times during the treatment in any one spot. This pressure point can correspond to a place in the body where life force energy is blocked, sluggish, or unbalanced. These blockages can sometimes move quite quickly when this pressure technique is applied. The patient may feel some sudden changes within, tingling sensations, becoming more relaxed, etc. The therapist may also feel things change, and even the atmosphere in the room might feel different in a very short period of time. If anything unpleasant is experienced, do not overstimulate this point; carry on with the normal treatment and things will settle down quickly. You can come back to the same point later or in another treatment.

In General

All the above techniques need to be practiced as much as possible on your own hands and feet, or on the feet of family or friends. Remember, you can do no harm with reflexology. It is a perfectly safe technique to use if you always follow the instructions and use a light massage technique until you have gained some experience.

There is some flexibility in the techniques used in reflexology, so as long as you learn the basics and do not stray too far from the orthodox treatment sequence.

You can then apply your own experience and creativity to improve the techniques as many reflexologists have done.

Reflexology is a very enjoyable therapy to practice and receive, and much fun can be had in learning and applying the techniques with friends and family. It is also fun to learn in a class with others or with a friend or partner where you can practice on each other—even at the same time! Children and babies love it, too.

The feet are really a whole new world to us. Most of us never really care about our feet, and we miss out on so much good health and improved quality of life because of this. If every family or group of friends had one member who knew reflexology, then the world would be a much healthier and, indeed, happier place to be.

4

Beginning a Treatment

Preparing for Patients

Before you can begin to see patients, there are some basic things you will need: a quiet treatment room or office area, a therapy couch or reclining chair, proper lighting, and good heating/cooling. These help to create a comfortable environment. There are lots of things you can do to make the treatment area feel more peaceful and welcoming. Some obvious pointers are the decor, using subtle colors and hanging pleasant pictures, placing flowers and plants around the room, and providing one or two comfy chairs to be used when you are talking to the client before and after the treatment. Crystals, aromatherapy burners, and relaxing music also can help create the right conditions conducive to successful treatments.

If you are working in other people's homes, you will have to make do and adapt accordingly. However, you can warn them beforehand that the treatment will be more effective if the room that you use is at least warm and quiet and that you should not be disturbed.

When setting up an appointment, give yourself a suitable period of uninterrupted time; a full treatment usually lasts between forty-five to fifty minutes (excluding the interview and setting up), depending on your experience and the patient's requirements. Try to avoid potential distractions by using a telephone answering machine, not answering the front door, and asking others not to disturb you during a treatment. It can also be useful to have a clock within view to keep track of time.

The First Treatment

If you are treating someone for the first time, put yourself in his or her position, and think about how you felt when you first received reflexology. Try to make the patient as welcome and comfortable as possible, without going overboard. Give the patient time to explain why he or she has come to see you and what benefits he or she hopes to gain from the treatment (i.e., expectations).

When a patient comes to you for the first time, you may need to explain to him or her exactly what reflexology is, how it works, and what the treatment entails. You should think about how you will explain these things. There is no reason to overload people with details, but it can be helpful to explain the basics, and it gives people confidence in your abilities if you obviously know what you are talking about.

However, judge every situation as you think best. Sometimes it may not seem appropriate as the patient may then be thinking about what might happen instead of just relaxing. Here are some examples of what you may wish to tell them, if it feels like the right thing to do:

- How long the treatment takes

- The treatment is done solely on the feet using the hands

- Demonstrate the basic hand techniques and let them know that they can just relax and enjoy it

- They may experience warmth in and around the body and/or coming from your hands; occasionally it may feel cool instead

- Tingling sensations may be felt in and around the body

- They may experience a sense of heaviness or lightness

- They may feel very relaxed or even sleepy; tell them it's okay to fall asleep

- They may want to talk, which is also fine

- They may sweat slightly or twitch at times; they may feel some "movement" within the body as they relax

- Their stomach may gurgle as their body relaxes

- Their throat may become dry, so have a glass of water at hand, and tissues for a runny nose

Explain to the patient that these are all natural reactions. Some people may have much deeper and more profound experiences and/or emotional releases, so an ability to listen and even a box of tissues may be useful. Try to be open and accept whatever arises, and trust that the patient will know consciously or subconsciously what he or she is ready to release and/or deal with. The more genuine trust and confidence you have in other's natural healing abilities, the easier it will be for those qualities to naturally arise within them. From the practitioner's side, developing this trust in the process of natural healing is part of your own healing and growth. It also creates the right atmosphere and conditions conducive to "ripening" the patient's own self-healing potential.

At the first treatment, you will also have to ask the patient to read and sign a disclaimer, although this is mainly important if you are practicing reflexology professionally and being paid for your services. Again, such topics will be covered in a practitioner's training course together with taking case notes and the client's personal details and medical history. (See chapter 6 for more information on educational practitioner courses.)

However, despite the best preparations, if you do not know how to treat your patient with respect, empathy, wisdom, and understanding, then you are fighting a losing battle. If the patient has confidence and faith in your abilities, and feels relaxed and able to talk freely without fear of judgment, then you can be assured that the barriers to healing will be gradually worn down. (See chapter 8 for more information on healing and dealing with patients.)

Pretreatment Practices

You will need to wash your hands before every treatment and possibly also the patient's feet. For the feet, you could use an antiseptic wipe or a damp cloth soaked in a bowl of warm water with some antiseptic diluted in it. Check the feet first for any cuts or sensitive areas that might sting from using the antiseptic.

If your hands are cold, warm them before starting the treatment. Obviously cold hands can be a shock to warm feet and hinder relaxation. You can warm your hands simply by tightly clenching your fists and then relaxing and shaking your hands. Do this several times until the blood begins to flow. Alternatively, you can put your hands in warm water for a few minutes and then repeat the clenching exercise.

From the patient's point of view, he or she needs to be physically and mentally relaxed to receive the greatest benefit from the treatment. The patient will normally lie down on a couch, or sit up in a chair, with his or her legs extended. The patient's bare feet should just dangle over the edge of the couch or a stool. It is important that the backs of the knees are supported in some way. Placing a flat pillow underneath them can help increase their comfort.

You as the therapist also has to be as comfortable as possible during the session, especially if you intend to do several successive treatments. A chair that supports the lower back is essential, and an erect but not stiff posture should be adopted so that your spine is not bent. Your back muscles will gradually strengthen with each treatment, and this will prevent wear and tear on the spine. It is also useful if the chair is on wheels, like an office chair, and preferably without armrests. This will enable you to move to around the area close to the feet, without having to stretch to reach things you may need. A small table, perhaps also on wheels, is useful to keep those items that you need close at hand.

It is also important to keep the feet warm at all times. As soon as the client has settled into a comfortable position, place a small towel over the feet. The towel can be prewarmed and wrapped around the feet, and tucked under the ankles, if this is comfortable for the patient. When you are ready to begin the treatment, unwrap the feet and place the towel around the foot you will not be treating to keep it warm.

Reading the Feet/Foot Inspection

When you inspect the feet, especially during the first treatment, you should be careful to notice certain conditions that are telltale signs of what areas that need to be concentrated on. When you look at the feet, what is the very first impression you get?

- Do they look tired, fat, thin, pale, red, deformed?

- What condition is the skin in? Is it dry, sweaty, cracked? Is it the same all over?

- When you touch and massage the feet, how do they react? Do they tense up or relax straight away? Do they feel stiff or lack vitality/energy?

- When you massage certain areas, do they feel, tense, puffy, inflamed, or lacking vitality?

- Can you feel anything under the skin like granules or grainy deposits? Do these break up under gentle massage or stubbornly remain?

All these indications tell you two things: the condition of the patient's body and the condition of the patient's mind. They also show you how healthy the client is as well as how unhealthy!

All these indications tell us that there is something going on inside the patient's body and/or mind that is being reflected in the feet. For example, hard skin on the top of the big toe might be found on someone who is prone to headaches. Soft or tender skin on the ball of the foot might be present in someone prone to chest infections or asthma. However, there are no rules as to what type of skin condition relates to what illness or physical weakness. You can only use them as a broad indication that some corresponding part of the body is in need of attention.

During the treatment you can spend a little longer on those areas of the feet that seem to be lacking vitality, have hard or tender skin, etc. You can also encourage the patient to gently massage these needy areas for a few minutes once or twice a day between treatments. You should also gently stress that if there is a strong detox reaction, the patient should then stop treatment until this passes. (See page 109 for a description of detox reactions.) You can also suggest to the patient to try to remove any hardened skin, soak his or her feet in warm water once a day, and perform a few simple exercises afterward. Such exercises might involve clockwise and counterclockwise ankle rotations, pointing the feet and holding for a few seconds, and then pulling them up to stretch the Achilles tendon. The patient can gently massage the feet as well but, again, only gently. Too much stimulation of the reflexes, especially in the first few weeks of treatment, can cause illness, sweating, increased urination, and other side effects (i.e., detox reactions). In rare cases, this can cause the client to cease treatment, believing it to be a source of further illness instead of helping his or her condition.

The feet don't lie. When patients expose their feet to you for treatment, they are unwittingly allowing you to see how they are physically and mentally. If you gradually learn to read the feet, you will become very good at understanding your clients. All the indications that the feet show you are valuable information that you need to assimilate and remember. If you are able to make notes on the state and condition of the feet during or before each treatment, and compare the improvements that take place with the improvements that take place in the patient's body and mind, you will be amazed at the obvious correlations.

You have to be careful not to alarm the patient with any signs or indications that you see. This can only depress or worry someone who might already be struggling to cope with a difficult illness. If in doubt, it is best to remain quiet. However, if you think that one of your patient's should seek medical advice, tell them. Also, what you see through the feet might not indicate an immediate problem, just an early warning sign.

Some reflexologists are also able to pick up, subconsciously, problems that the patient has, right from the first treatment. It can be a little like having your fortune told. Again, palm reading through the soles of the feet is not part of traditional reflexology, but if you naturally develop such skills, they can be used wisely or sparingly to help others who are open to such help.

It is also good practice to check the feet thoroughly for any localized medical conditions. It is useful to tell the patient what you are doing as you inspect each foot and between each toe. Be sure to make notes about what you find on a case study sheet. It is rare to find a pair of feet where you have to refuse treatment due to a medical condition that can be transmitted by touch to other patients. You can simply avoid the infected area or wear medical-grade rubber gloves. The following are some of the common conditions you may come across:

Athlete's foot: A fungal infection that usually forms between the toes but in serious cases can spread further. It is characterized by loose, flaking skin, and itching and irritation. It is easily transmitted to others.

Toenail problems: These can include fungal infections (which can be transmitted to others), and involuted, ingrown, or thickened toenails.

Corns and calluses: These are thickened, hardened layers of skin. Corns often appear as raised bumps while calluses can vary in size and shape.

Bunions: These are painful inflammations of the bursa at the base of the big toe, causing it to bend toward the next toe.

Heel calluses, spurs, and fissures: A callus is a hard, thick area of skin. A spur is a sharp projection of bone. A fissure is a cleft-like defect in the skin.

High arches and flatfeet: Flatfeet is the absence of an arch in the foot.

Plantar warts/verucas: Plantar warts appear on the sole of the foot. The wart virus can be spread by touch.

Gout: This is a form of arthritis caused by the build-up of too much uric acid in the blood, which then becomes deposited around the joints, usually at the base of the big toe, causing swelling and redness.

Eczema: These are typically patches of dry, reddened, swollen, and/or itchy skin.

Plantar digital neuritis: This is the inflammation of the nerves affecting the toes, usually occurring in women only.

A good medical textbook will give detailed descriptions and pictures of these conditions. Taking reflexology courses will also cover these and other medical conditions as well. It is worth looking them up so that you know what to expect. Obviously, most patients will know what foot problems they have and will usually tell you before the first treatment. If you do not want to treat someone, with for example verucas, then simply ask the patient to seek medical advice and to come and see you when he or she has been successfully treated.

Some foot problems like arthritis will mean you will have to be especially gentle so as not to cause discomfort during the treatment. It is most important that a patient's treatment is comfortable and relaxing. Patients will not be able to relax if they expect pain, so reassure clients that you will be gentle and ask them to let you know if and where there is any discomfort. Again, you can make notes about each patient to remind you for future treatments.

There is one field of thought that suggests foot deformities caused by uncomfortable shoes contribute to poor health. This might be because the reflexes and meridians in the feet are distorted and distressed, and this has a corresponding effect on the relevant organs and systems of the body. In such cases, you can recommend that your client wear more comfortable footwear whenever possible, and that this will help the body greatly. Also walking barefoot in a warm environment as much as is practical or possible is a good way to gradually reshape the feet into their normal position, if the damage is not too well established.

Once you are satisfied with the foot inspection, the next step is to loosen and relax the feet with a few simple stretching and rotating exercises—warming up the feet. This also helps the patient to relax and gain confidence in you as a therapist before the treatment begins.

Warming Up the Feet

The following movements for stretching and relaxing the feet should always used at the beginning of a treatment. They help the client relax physically and mentally, they warm the feet, and also help the therapist prepare mentally and physically. Some reflexologists also use these techniques during and after a treatment. They help to keep the foot relaxed and ensure a free flow of life force energy around the body.

The sequence you choose to relax the feet is not too important. The way the various movements are presented is an effective sequence, but your experience may show you otherwise. If you think of some new movements, try them on yourself or a friend first to see if they are comfortable and useful. Again, it is important to gain some experience in giving and receiving these warm-up movements.

It is also worth bearing in mind that the feet of patients on their first treatment will be stiffer and might need more gentle treatment and no overstretching. You could perform more stretching movements throughout the main part of the treatment to keep the feet supple.

Always begin gently; then there is no fear of injury. As always, be especially careful with sensitive, "sick," or "new" feet (i.e., new patients). Some of the warm-up exercises can be used throughout the rest of the treatment and can form part of the treatment. In fact, if you only have a short amount of time, say ten to fifteen minutes, they can be used to give a short treatment. For example, they could be practiced on someone who has just come home from work to help wind down, or first thing in the morning to help wake up. This is an excellent method for relaxing and destressing anyone in only a short amount of time.

Stretching and Squeezing the Achilles Tendon

Following Figure 16, support the heel in the palm of one hand and place the palm of the other hand over the ball of the foot. Gently push the ball of the foot away from you, using only minimal pressure at first. Then pull the foot toward you, your fingers gently wrapped around the top of the foot. Make sure that you do not

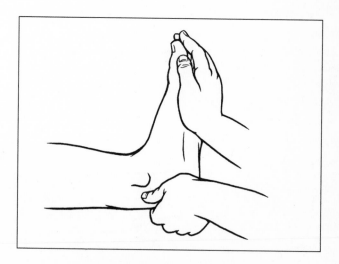

Figure 16: *Achilles tendon stretch*

bend the toes forward. Repeat this procedure three or four times. Each time you will be able to push and pull a little farther as the tendon stretches. As you stretch the tendon, gently squeeze it with the supporting hand. Repeat on the other foot, reversing the hands.

Rotating the Foot

Following Figure 17, support the heel by cupping it in the palm of one hand. With your other hand, gently grab the patient's toes, your thumb on the ball of the foot. Begin to rotate the foot clockwise for three or four rotations, then counterclockwise. The rotations should be as wide as possible. Again, judge this by how far the

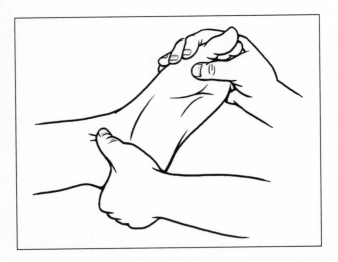

Figure 17: *Rotating the foot*

foot naturally moves without excessively stretching it. The ankle bones may "crack" as they are rotated and loosened. This is good, so long as the patient is not uncomfortable or concerned. Repeat on the other foot.

Loosening the Ankles

Following Figure 18, use the side of each hand to grip the naturally concave area below the ankle bone. Move your hands back and forth in opposite directions. The foot will wobble from side to side as you do this, and it is the momentum of this wobbling that helps to loosen the ankle. If the movement is too slow, it will not work as effectively.

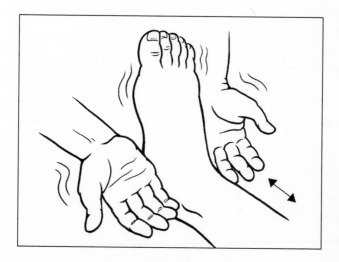

Figure 18: Loosening the ankles

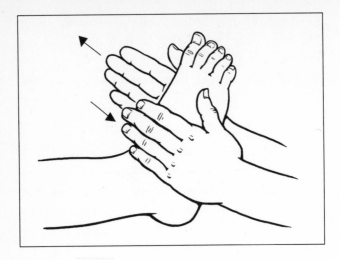

Figure 19: *Loosening the foot*

Loosening the Foot

Following Figure 19, gently "grip" the sides of the foot with your palms. Bring one palm toward you while "pushing" the other palm away from you until some resistance is met. Then reverse the movement. This gently stretches and loosens the foot. Repeat this motion several times. If the patient remains comfortable, you can increase the speed and vigor of the movement. Repeat on the other foot.

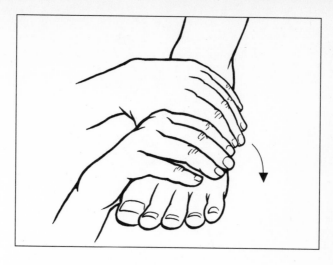

Figure 20: *Gently twisting the foot (spinal twist)*

Spinal Twist

This has a similar effect as loosening the foot and can be used instead of or with that exercise. It also works on the spine reflex. Following Figure 20, grab the inner side of the foot with both hands, your thumbs on the sole of the foot and fingers on top. Begin a gentle rotating motion, first one way and then the other. This is not a wringing motion! Both hands should work in the same direction. In this position, you can also "bend" the foot, as if breaking some bread in half. Again, the motion is slow and gentle, never using force or strong pressure as this only causes discomfort.

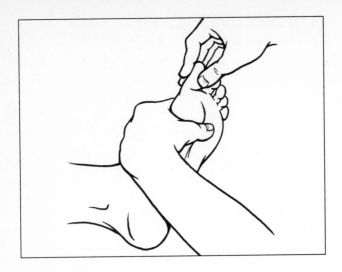

Figure 21: *Rotating and pulling the toe*

Rotating and Pulling the Toes

Following Figure 21, support the foot with the basic support hold. With your thumb and index finger (and second finger, if necessary) grab the big toe near the base. The thumb will be under the toe and the finger on the top. With this gentle grip, begin to rotate the toe one way and then the other for about three rotations, both ways. Repeat this with each toe.

To gently pull the toe to help release tension, slowly relax your grip and let the thumb and finger slide slowly up the toe to the tip. At the tip, give a gentle pinch, but not if the client's toes are particularly sensitive, or if there is an ingrown toenail or some other ailment. Sometimes there might be a case for holding the tip of each toe as a pressure hold, as this will reflex to all the zones in the body. This might suit some clients but not others, and with experience you will learn when to use this and at what point in the treatment.

Wringing the Foot

Following Figure 22, gently grab the top of the foot with both hands. Begin a wringing action, the hands gently but firmly twisting the foot in opposite directions. Be careful not to stretch the skin! Only a firm, slow action is needed. Twist in opposite directions two or three times, beginning at the base of the foot and moving the hands toward the toes. The foot will be more flexible

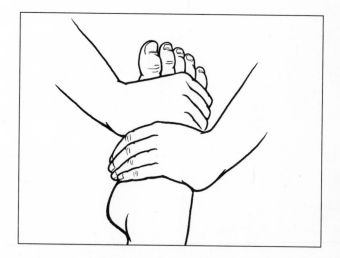

Figure 22: *Wringing the foot*

nearer to the toes. Before doing this exercise, some practitioners like to use the same hand hold to squeeze the foot from the heel to the toes, as this gently pushes the bones together and helps the muscles relax more.

Solar Plexus Press

To find the solar plexus point, squeeze the sides of the foot together. A natural crease will appear toward the center of the sole, just below the ball of the foot. The solar plexus reflex area is located in the depression at the center of this crease. Place your thumb on the solar plexus reflex, with the fingers wrapped around the front of each foot. (See Figure 23.) Do both feet at the

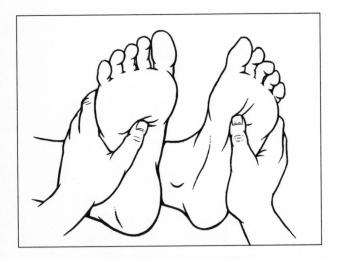

Figure 23: *Solar plexus press*

same time. As the patient inhales, apply pressure by pushing the thumbs into the sole of the foot. The foot will move back under the pressure. Do not use the fingers to squeeze the foot. As the patient exhales, release the pressure and allow the feet to move back toward you. Repeat this three or four times in time with the patient's breathing.

Some reflexologists only use this exercise as a warm-down after the treatment, and some actually ask the patient to breathe more deeply and hold the breath for a few seconds while applying the pressure on the reflex and then exhaling on the release. Again this is a matter of personal preference; experience and intuition will show you the way.

General Warm-Up Advice

There are other techniques used to relax the foot, like simply rhythmically stroking the top of the foot from the ankle to the toes, using one hand after another. Another is to support the top of the foot with one hand while gently but firmly pushing the flat side of a clenched fist into the base of the foot, again working from the ball of the foot down to the heel. (See Figure 24, page 72.) You can try turning the fist at the same time in a sort of gentle kneading movement. Also try gently squeezing the foot from top to bottom and giving a general gentle massage using the fingers and thumbs.

Reflexologists tend to develop their own style of warm-up procedures, so try the above exercises on a few friends to see what they like and to see what you

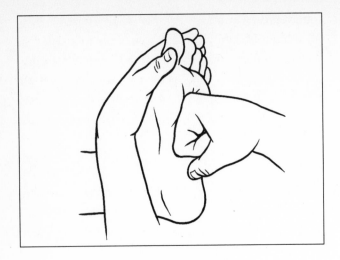

Figure 24: Fist press

feel is most helpful. But don't get stuck in a rut with one set of techniques. With experience, you will get to know which patients like which kind of warm-up and how much pressure to apply. Also, don't be too light with your touch techniques. Sometimes an almost vigorous warm-up and a firm touch during the treatment might really suit a particular patient. Again, experience and confidence will be your guides.

Self-Treatment

Some books go into detail about the various techniques of self-treatment. If you have a choice, it is always far better to receive a reflexology treatment from someone else, even a novice, than to treat yourself. If there is no one you can turn to, then by all means, treat yourself. The main reason why self-treatment is inferior is the lack of comfort and inability to relax during treatment.

To treat the sole of your foot, you will have to lift one foot onto the thigh of the other leg to reach it, and this can be uncomfortable for any length of time, especially if you have joint or back problems. If you want to persevere with self-treatment, try ten minutes of reflexology on each foot, every day for a week. Use the different techniques described in this book. As long as you give the whole foot a thorough going-over, either using the fingers, thumbs, knuckles, palms, or fists, then your self-treatment will be effective.

After the first week, cut the treatments down to every other day, then every third day in the third week, then once or twice a week thereafter. You may experience a big improvement in your state of physical and mental health. Keep the treatments up and this should continue.

Foot Note

As mentioned before, there is no substitute for practice and experience to become an accomplished reflexologist. At the beginning, it may seem that there is too much to learn, but if you learn a little at a time and practice a little every day, you will easily be able to complete your first full treatment within a few weeks, even before if you apply more effort. Obviously you will not be able to practice professionally without completing an appropriate course of study, but you will be able to bring great benefit to friends and family who will be lining up to take advantage of your new-found skills. There is a great sense of satisfaction and joy in seeing the results of a good treatment. This sense of accomplishment that you are doing something creative and meaningful with your time can be the fuel to encourage you to improve and advance your skills further.

You are now ready to begin the main part of the treatment.

5

The Main Treatment

A full treatment is made up of individual sections that, through the foot reflexes, treat particular areas or systems of the body, like the head, heart and lungs, spine, lymphatic system, and so on. Don't worry if you do not know in detail what some of these physiological systems do since brief explanations are given in chapter 2 to refer to. You can also study more in-depth texts on human anatomy and physiology as you progress.

Once you have completed all your treatment preparations, taken your client's details, explained how the treatment works, and completed the warm-up exercises, you can move on to the main part of the treatment.

There are several schools of thought concerning the order in which the various reflexes should be treated. What follows is one of the most well-known and widely used. But that does not mean it is necessarily any more effective than others. Once you have mastered these basics and gained experience, you can look at other schools of thought and decide for yourself what to use and what to discard.

It is easier to learn the reflexes for each body system while also learning about the system itself, so it is worth referring regularly to the illustrations and explanations in chapter 2. You will also need to remind yourself of where the more intricate reflexes are located.

As some of the reflexes for different physiological systems overlap, you can make changes to the sequence of treatment to make it slightly quicker and more efficient but just as effective. But it is important to learn the basics well before you do this.

As a general rule, if you cover all of the reflexes in one treatment, then this is the main requirement. In the beginning, if you get the order wrong or forget to complete the sequence of reflexes for a system, you can just add them on at the end of the treatment, or at an appropriate point midsession.

Treatment Techniques

These are the techniques for a full treatment. Remember to refer back to the detailed illustrations in chapter 2 showing the location of each reflex with its associated body part or function. There are some specific techniques for treating particular reflexes. Generally, as long as you cover all the reflexes in one section of the treatment, there is no specific order that is more effective than another. During your first few treatments, you are bound to forget to treat some reflexes, and this is fine, no harm can be done. If you learn each section methodically, within a few weeks you will be able to give a full treatment without referring to the book. This is a great feeling and shows that you are really deepening your knowledge, understanding, and experience of reflexology.

In fact, the sooner you can give treatments without referring to the book, the better. You can then begin to really tune in to the patient and develop your own style of reflexology. It is not a race, but the quicker you learn the basics, the quicker you can relax and start to listen to what the patient needs and also develop your own intuitive healing abilities. If you have or develop a genuine wish to help others without a strong sense of self-importance or pride as a healer, then you will definitely become an accomplished reflexologist and a real source of help to others.

As with most of the various treatments where the same reflexes exist on both feet, begin with one foot (usually the patient's right foot) and then treat the same reflex on the other foot. Some reflexologists prefer to treat one foot almost completely while keeping the other warmly but loosely wrapped up in a small towel. Again, with experience, you can decide which is more effective.

All the feet you treat will be a slightly different size and shape, so the reflexes will also vary slightly in location. The general shape of the foot is the clue to locating them, and the illustrations given throughout this book are an accurate guide on which to base your treatments.

Toes/Head and Neck

The toe reflexes correlate to the head and neck area of the body. (Refer to the reflex chart in Figure 2, page 18.) Concentrating on the very tip of each toe, you can treat the sinus reflexes. You can do this by simply using the nibbling or thumb walking massage explained in chapter 3, pages 44–45.

Following Figure 25, support the foot with one hand, using the basic foot support hold, with the thumb supporting the bottom of the toe to be worked on. Then begin using the walking massage with your other thumb on the very tip of each toe. Be sure not to bend the toe.

The same walking massage technique can be used to treat the front and back of each toe. Following Figure 26, support the foot using the basic foot support hold. Then use the thumb and index finger to simultaneously massage and support the front and back of each toe. (The front of the toes can be worked on using the index finger while the thumb supports the back of the toe and vice versa.) Remember that the toes are often quite sensitive, especially between the toes, so a gentle touch is important.

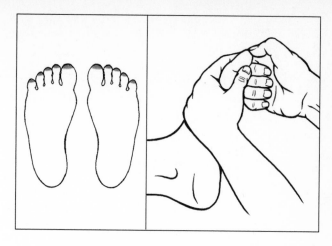

Figure 25: *Locating and treating the reflexes
on the tips of the toes (sinuses)*

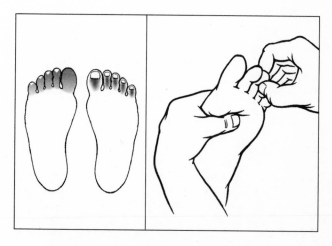

Figure 26: *Locating and treating the reflexes
on the front and back of the toes*

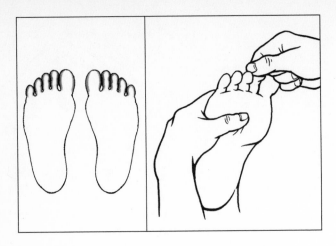

Figure 27: *Locating and treating the reflexes on the sides of the toes*

The side of each toe can be treated the same as the front and back by using the index finger to massage each toe gently from the top to the bottom. (See Figure 27.)

Do not skimp on massaging the toes. They are at least as important as the rest of the foot. In acupuncture it is known that the six main meridians, or energy channels, are all stimulated by massaging the feet, especially the toes.

By using these techniques thoroughly, you will have covered nearly all the main reflexes for the head and neck. By referring back to the reflex chart (Figure 2, page 18), you will see that there are many important areas treated, especially those relating to the brain, that

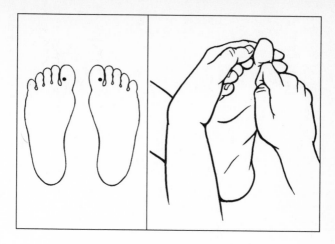

Figure 28: *Locating and treating the pituitary reflex on the bottom on the foot*

you may find the patient is already quite relaxed and that some healing energy is really starting to flow.

One of these important reflexes is the pituitary gland. It is found within the brain reflex on the big toe. (See Figure 28.) It will take a little experience to find it, and the best way to do this is to visually locate the center of the spiral on the bottom of the big toe. (See reflex chart Figure 2, page 18.) To massage, use the knuckle of your index finger and press on the reflex, rotate, and lift. (See Figure 28.) If you have located it correctly, the patient will feel a sharp, little pain in the toe. Do not cause too much pain by overstimulating it. Make sure to do this on both big toes.

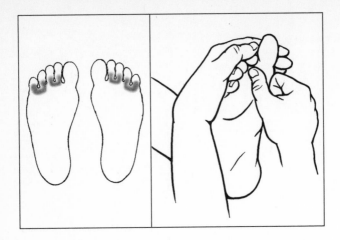

Figure 29: *Locating and treating the reflexes on the base of the toes on the bottom of the foot (eyes and ears)*

Move on to the areas just below the base of each toe on the bottom of the foot. (See Figure 29.) Use the thumb to massage these reflexes relating to the eyes and ears (refer to reflex chart Figure 2, page 18). You can use the thumb of the supporting hand to bend the toes slightly forward, thus creating a shelf-like area on which to work. Work in a horizontal line across the ball of the foot, from the outside of the foot in.

The final reflexes to treat in the toe area are the upper lymphatic reflexes at the base of the toes on the top of the foot. They are stimulated using the single finger massage technique (refer to Figure 13, page 47).

Following Figure 30, support the foot by gently grabbing the foot so your palm is cupping the sole of

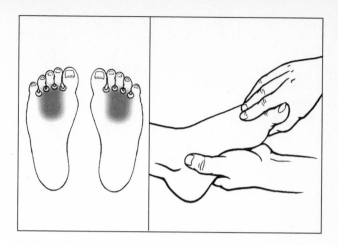

Figure 30: *Locating and treating the reflexes on the base of the toes on top of the foot (upper lymphatic system)*

the foot and your thumb is near the inner ankle bone. Using your index finger on your other hand, work the reflex area (shaded area shown in Figure 30) in vertical lines, from the toes toward the heel. You especially want to concentrate on the area between the foot bones. You will feel the bones move apart slightly as you apply pressure. Again, these areas might be sensitive, so be careful not to apply too much pressure during the patient's first or second treatment.

This is also a good time to treat the whole top of the foot, if you wish, by simply using the same technique to continue the massage up to the lymphatic reflexes on the ankle. (See reflex chart Figure 6, page 30). Do not go down the side of the foot as these areas are covered

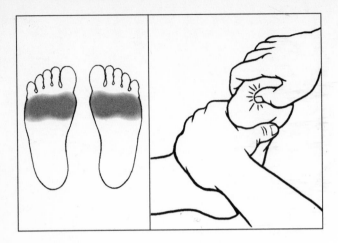

Figure 31: *Locating and treating the reflexes on the ball of the foot (heart, lung, and bronchi)*

later. This whole area helps the lymphatic system, as well as stimulate and relax many other bodily functions and systems.

Ball of the Foot/Thoracic Region

There are some major organs and glands located in this area. Many medical conditions relating to the heart, lungs, and thyroid, for example, respond well to treating these reflexes. (See reflex chart Figure 3, page 21.)

Following Figure 31, support the top of the foot with one hand while using the thumb walking technique with the other hand to massage the reflexes. The shaded area in Figure 31 denotes the heart, lung, and

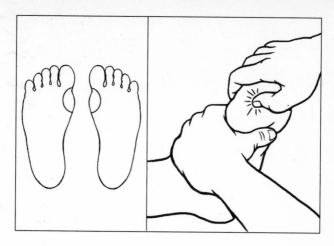

Figure 32: *Locating and treating the reflexes on the ball of the foot (thyroid, parathyroid, and neck)*

bronchial reflexes. Since this area is often covered by toughened skin, as it takes the whole weight of the body when we walk, you might have to apply a little more pressure than usual. Work in vertical lines, from bottom to top or from left to right, using your right and then left thumb. Alternatively, you can work in diagonal lines one way and then the other. The main goal is to cover the whole area.

Figure 32 shows the location of the thyroid, parathyroid, and the base of the neck reflexes. Support the foot by gently grabbing the inside of the foot, the thumb just below the ball of the foot. Use the thumb walking massage technique to massage the semicircular line shown in Figure 32 upward, from the ball of the

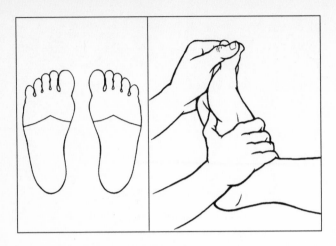

Figure 33: *Locating and treating the reflexes
on the ball of the foot (diaphragm)*

foot to the base of the big toe. Repeat this two or three times. Then cover the area between this line and the inside of the foot again by using vertical, diagonal, or horizontal lines. Again, this may be a sensitive area, so proceed with caution on a new patient.

The diaphragm reflex is located directly below the ball of the foot. It is the imaginary line separating the ball of the foot from the arch. Figure 33 shows this line of a typical diaphragm reflex, although as with all reflexes they are slightly different from patient to patient. (Also see reflex chart Figure 3, page 21.)

Following Figure 33, the support hand holds the toes and pushes them back slightly, while bringing the foot slightly toward you. Use your other thumb to work along the line of the diaphragm, from the outside in. Work in very short vertical or diagonal lines, or just horizontally in two or three lines close together, to cover the diaphragm reflex area.

Arch of the Foot/Abdominal Area

Referring back to the reflex chart in Figure 4, page 24, you will see that most of the reflexes for the digestive system are located in the arch of the foot. This area is also the most complicated in terms of the number of reflexes and the way they often overlap. Some reflexology books present complicated methods for treating each reflex in a specific order. This can be very effective, but there is no research or anecdotal evidence to suggest it is any more effective than using a simple horizontal, vertical, and/or diagonal thumb walking technique to cover the area from top to bottom. Alternatively, a simple compromise can take the best from the complicated system and simple system, as follows below.

Also, remember that the arch area can be more sensitive to touch, so this area will require less pressure to stimulate the reflexes.

The shaded area in Figure 34, page 88, shows the location of the liver reflex. Being such a large organ, the liver reflex takes up a substantial area on the bottom of the patient's right foot (the liver organ is also located on the right side of the body). To massage the reflex, use your right hand to hold the upper part of the foot as support and your left thumb as the massage tool. (See

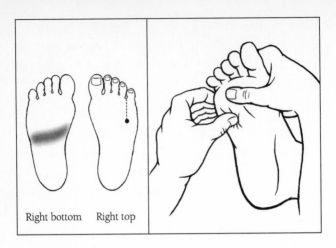

Right bottom   Right top

Figure 34: *Locating and treating the liver and gall bladder reflexes*

Figure 34.) Work from top to bottom and left to right, in horizontal or diagonal lines. As you work down the liver reflex, you will also begin to work the stomach, pancreas, and duodenum reflexes as they overlap this area.

Once you have worked the liver, you should now locate the gall bladder reflex, also on the bottom of the right foot. One way to locate it is to run your finger down the top of the foot, between the fourth and fifth toes. About 2 inches down, you will find a small dip or indentation. (See Figure 34.) Be gentle as this may be sensitive.

Now locate this same position on the bottom of the foot, and this will be the gall bladder reflex. You can

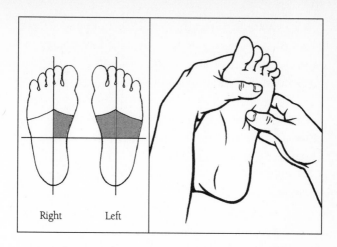

Figure 35: *Locating and treating the upper abdominal area reflexes (stomach, pancreas, duodenum, and spleen)*

press and massage it in a circular motion, or just gently press and hold for five to ten seconds. Some reflexologists like to use the left finger and thumb to press and hold the top and bottom of the foot at the same time. Also, some reflexologists do not treat the gall bladder separately at all but feel that simply working the liver is enough.

The next important reflexes in the abdominal area are the stomach, pancreas, duodenum, and spleen. (Refer to reflex chart in Figure 4, page 24.) The shaded areas in Figure 35 show what needs to be covered to treat them effectively, which is basically the inside arch area. It is also important to avoid the liver reflex area, as overstimulating the reflexes is never beneficial.

Start with the patient's right foot. In Figure 35, the shaded right half of the bottom right foot covers the stomach, pancreas, and duodenum reflexes. Grab the upper part of the foot with your right hand in the basic support hold. Then use your left thumb to work the area, moving away from the midpoint (where the lines intersect), and then back toward it with the right thumb, if you want to.

Now move to the patient's left foot, reversing your hand positions. Figure 35 shows the shaded left half of the bottom left foot that you will start working on. Use your right thumb to treat the reflex areas for the stomach, pancreas, duodenum, and spleen, moving in toward the midpoint. Then change hand positions, working with the left thumb up to the midpoint.

Now treat the right half of the bottom left foot. This area, shown in Figure 35, covers part of the stomach, spleen, and part of the colon. Use your left thumb to work toward the outside of the foot. Then switch hands/thumbs and work toward the midpoint.

As the shaded areas in Figure 36 show, the lower part of the arch of the foot includes the reflexes for the small intestine, ileo-caecal valve, appendix, and large intestine. (Also refer to reflex chart Figure 4, page 24, for the specific locations of the reflexes.) The best way to treat these areas is in the general direction in which the intestines work.

Start with the patient's right foot. Support the foot with your right hand. Begin working the small intestine with your left thumb, moving from left to right in

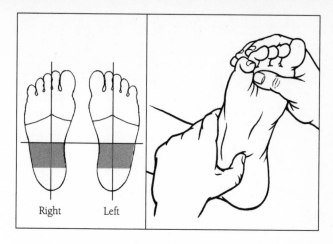

Figure 36: *Locating and treating the lower abdominal area reflexes (intestines and appendix)*

horizontal lines. You can work across this area from top to bottom as well.

Now work the small intestine reflex on the patient's left foot, changing hand positions accordingly.

Once this is complete, return to the patient's right foot to begin working the large intestine/colon, from the bottom left-hand corner of this area. At this point you will also stimulate the ileo-caecal valve reflex, which you can press and hold for a few seconds before beginning to work up and across on the large intestine/colon reflex.

Now move back to the patient's left foot. Continue with the left thumb until we reach the far right of the

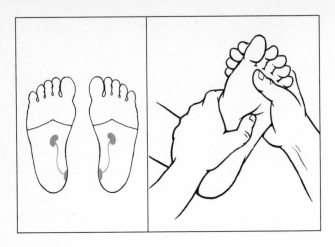

Figure 37: *Locating and treating the kidneys,
adrenals, ureter, and bladder reflexes*

foot (from the therapist's perspective). Then switch
hands, using the right thumb to work down the
remaining area of the reflex, down to the sigmoid flexure and anus.

The remaining reflexes to be covered in the arch
area are for the urinary system, and these include the
kidneys, adrenals, ureter, and bladder. Most of these
reflexes will have already been stimulated if you have
followed the previous instructions carefully. However,
most reflexologists like to work them again and more
accurately with the following method. If you are worried about overstimulation, use a lighter touch when
you cover these areas in previous sections and again
when treating them specifically.

Figure 37 shows the reflexes for the kidneys, adrenals, ureter, and bladder. (See also the reflex chart in Figure 4, page 24.) The adrenals are located directly on the kidneys so both can be treated at the same time. The best way to locate the kidneys/adrenals is first to find the solar plexus reflex (see Figure 23, page 70) and then about one-thumb width (about the size of the patient's thumb) below this is the kidney reflex.

You will work the patient's right kidney first and then the left kidney, then move on to the right and left ureter, and finally the right and left bladder. The easiest way to work these areas is by using your right thumb on the patient's right foot and your left thumb on the patient's left foot.

To begin, use the basic support hold to support the foot. Alternatively, you can try using your left thumb to work the kidney down to the top of the bladder on the patient's right foot and then your right thumb works the bladder and vice versa for the other foot. Some reflexologists like to treat all these reflexes on one foot at a time; either way is effective.

Figure 38, page 94, shows how the bladder reflex curves around the inside of the foot. It can appear like an area of "slack," limp, or puffy skin. It can also be sensitive, so a light touch should be used initially.

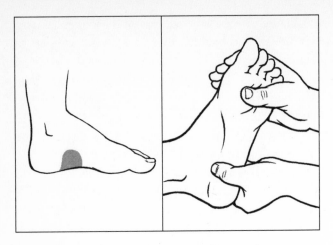

Figure 38: *Locating and treating the bladder reflex*
on the inside of the foot

Heel/Pelvic Area

This part of the foot often has the toughest skin so a little more pressure is required. The areas to be worked
are shown in Figure 39. (Also see the reflex chart in Figure 5, page 29.) The knuckle press technique (see Figure 15, page 48) is used to reach the reflexes beneath
the hardened layer of skin. In the cases of elderly, sick,
or disabled people, the skin may be softer on the heel so
the regular thumb walking technique can be used instead, as the knuckle massage may cause discomfort.
Also, the heel area may be especially sensitive in people
with a physical problem in the corresponding pelvic
region. Again, you can work from side to side or top to
bottom to cover this area.

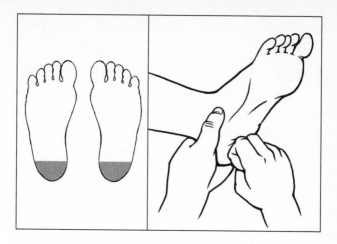

Figure 39: *Locating and treating the heel reflexes (pelvic area)*

Ankles/Reproductive Organs

The reflexes for all the reproductive organs are located in the ankle area. (Refer to reflex chart in Figure 6, page 30.) These can often be quite sensitive, so a gentle touch is required, especially for the first few treatments.

The top foot illustration in Figure 40, page 97, shows the ovaries and testes reflex, which is found on the outside of the foot, also about midway between the ankle bone and the top of the heel.

The bottom foot illustration in Figure 40 shows the reflexes for the uterus and prostate, which are found on the inside of the foot, about midway between the ankle bone and the top of the heel.

To begin, work the prostate/uterus reflex on the inside of the patient's left foot. Support the foot with your right hand and use your left thumb to massage the reflex. (See Figure 40.) Then simply reverse hands to treat the ovaries/testes reflex on the outside of the foot. Then move on to the inside of the patient's right foot, again starting with the prostate/uterus reflex.

As Figure 41 shows, the fallopian tubes and vas deferens reflexes are found on top of the ankles, running from the inner ankle bone to the outer one. (Again, refer to reflex chart Figure 6, page 30.) They can be worked simultaneously using the index and second fingers of both hands, working from the inner and outer ankle bones toward the center. (See Figure 41.) Your thumbs should be grabbing the ball of the foot, helping to support the foot. Alternatively, you can work one side and then the other, just use the other hand to support the foot by cupping the heel or grabbing the top of the foot.

Inner Foot/Spine

The spine reflex runs up the inner aspect of the foot from the top of the heel to the base of the big toe, where the neck reflex begins. (See Figure 42, page 98, and also the reflex charts in Figures 7 and 8, pages 32–33.) Since it is such an important part of the nervous system, treating this reflex will have a beneficial effect on the whole body.

The spinal twist used in the warm-up exercises can again be used here to begin treating this area. (See Figure 20, page 67.)

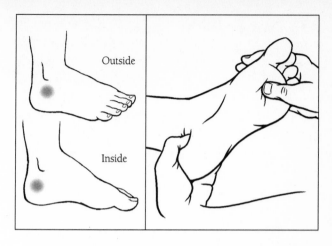

Figure 40: *Locating and treating the inner and outer ankle reflexes (reproductive organs)*

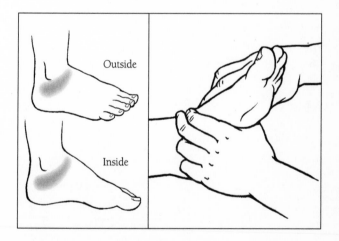

Figure 41: *Locating and treating the top of the ankle reflexes (fallopian tubes and vas deferens)*

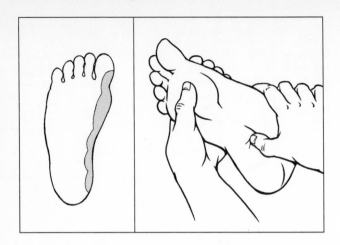

Figure 42: *Treating the inner foot*
reflexes (spine and neck)

Then, following Figure 42, use the basic thumb walking technique to begin massaging at the top of the heel, working your way up toward the big toe, following the line of the reflex. This reflex is actually split, with the left side of the spine located on the inside of the patient's left foot and the right side of the spine located on the inside of the right foot. You can work each foot several times, working slightly to the left/ right of the main reflex to ensure you have covered it completely.

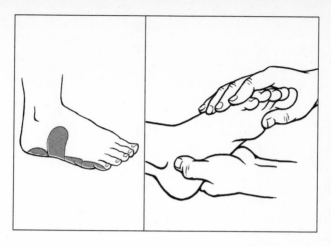

Figure 43: *Locating and treating the outer foot reflexes (knees, hips, arms)*

Outer Foot/Outer Body

Figure 43 shows the outer aspect of the patient's right foot, revealing the reflexes for the knees, hips, elbows, and shoulders. The hip reflex is the largest shaded area while the shoulder reflex is located by the little toe. (Refer also to reflex chart Figure 9, page 35.)

Starting with the patient's right foot, use your right hand to support the top of the foot. Then use your left hand to work these reflexes, from toe to heel, with the thumb walking technique. Switch hands to treat the other foot.

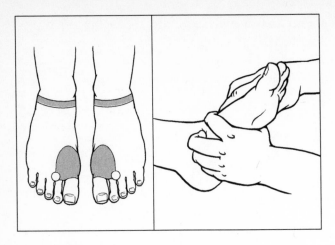

Figure 44: *Locating and treating the top of the foot reflexes (chest and circulation)*

Top of the Foot/Chest and Circulation

Figure 44 shows the reflexes that affect the chest area and circulation to be treated on top of the foot. (Also see reflex chart Figure 10, page 36.) Near the beginning of the treatment, you covered this area when treating the upper lymphatics, so only a light touch is now required to prevent overstimulation. You can work some reflexes a little more vigorously if there is a specific problem in the corresponding area of the body.

You can work the top of the foot gently using three or four fingers of each hand to cover the whole area, from the base of the toes to the ankles. When you reach the ankle bones, you can gently massage the

inner and outer bones in a circular motion simultaneously. Then repeat the procedure once or twice.

Warming Down

The last part of a treatment is also the first of the warm-
down techniques. The others in this sequence can include some of the gentler warm-up techniques and a
general light massage over the whole foot. You will develop your own techniques in time; ones that are simply relaxing are the best. As well as being the perfect
conclusion to the treatment, they give the client a
subtle hint that the treatment is nearly over.

Ending the Treatment

Often the best way to end a treatment is to use the
solar plexus press technique explained in chapter 4.
While relaxing, this also helps to wake the client up if
they are asleep or drowsy. If the patient is still asleep,
simply squeeze the feet gently, or touch the patient on
the shoulder. Do allow them plenty of time to come
around before sitting or standing up. There is no rush,
and the last thing you want to do is hurry the patient
out and the next one in!

Once the treatment is complete, you can touch
the person's shoulder if he or she is deeply relaxed
and not aware that the treatment is over and tell them
to sit up slowly when they are ready, then stand up
slowly. Try to give the patient time to talk and collect

him or herself after the treatment. Offer some refreshments as a little sugar and liquid can help people become "grounded" and alert after a very relaxing treatment. This is especially important if the patient has to drive home.

Remember that some people can become physically and mentally energized by a reflexology treatment while others are left feeling relaxed and ready to unwind. Don't take either as a good or a bad sign, as the good results of a treatment can take days to become apparent.

If you are doing several successive treatments give yourself a few minutes rest between each treatment, and set a mental intention to relax and recharge yourself. Don't take on too much too soon. In the beginning, just do a few treatments per week. This will give you time to build up your strength, stamina, and concentration. If you find that you are drained after a treatment, ask yourself if you are too tense during the treatment or if you are using too much pressure. Remember, a gentle touch is usually all that is required. You are not forcing the patient to get better, just gently encouraging good health to arise.

6

Practical Advice

Additional Benefits of Reflexology

Typical reactions during and after a reflexology treatment are the following:

- Increased energy
- Inner peace and a feeling of warmth within and/or around the body
- Gentle tingling sensations, especially in the hands which may also feel hot
- A sense of energy flowing in and/or around the body
- Clearer senses
- Less stress and emotional problems
- Improved physical health

- Increased ability to deal positively with stressful situations
- Increased clarity of mind and deeper intuitive or inner wisdom
- A sense of "coming home" and of being in touch with "the flow" of life
- Deepening of spiritual awareness and experiences (e.g., seeing or sensing auras, energy, colors, etc.)
- A general feeling of being more whole, healthy, and happy; a more complete sense of self

Everyone is different. Some people may feel nothing during a treatment and this is also normal! Reflexology works in the way that we need it as individuals, so you should not expect any two people to react in the same way, even when they have the same illness.

Educational Courses and Insurance

Can you really learn reflexology from a book? Yes! In fact, you can become quite an accomplished practitioner simply through reading books, practicing regularly, and receiving treatments from a fully qualified reflexologist (to experience how other healers work). This is ideal if you simply wish to treat yourself, friends, and family.

However, if you wish to practice professionally, you will need to pursue a recognized course of study and obtain the relevant qualifications. This is as much for your own benefit as for the people you will be treating. There are many reflexology courses available today as it is a well-respected and widely known form of complementary therapy.

You will also need to obtain professional indemnity insurance, so you will again need a recognized qualification for this.

Many people who take reflexology courses and other complementary therapies have no intention of practicing professionally but simply wish to be able to treat friends and family. The courses are not difficult and are generally very interesting, enjoyable, and well-structured so that anyone can complete them, feeling confident in their ability to treat others. You will also meet many people of like mind, and benefit from the company and sharing of ideas about your chosen therapy.

If you are simply learning from a book for your own pleasure, or wishing to start a course soon, there is no reason why you cannot start practicing the basic techniques explained in this book right away. You cannot cause harm and the more hands-on experience you can get, the better you will become. You should only practice on those you know well and never make any claims that you can cure any kind of illness. When friends and family experience the pleasure and positive results of a good treatment, then you will have a long queue of willing patients beating a path to your door!

Learning reflexology can be great fun, and when you begin to get good results, this can encourage you to learn more and help hone your skills to perfection. There is a real sense of accomplishment and satisfaction from seeing the benefits others derive from your new-found skills. (For a list of reflexology organizations, visit Llewellyn.com for a link to the author's website.)

The Healing Therapist

From the therapist's point of view, it is important to have a relaxed state of mind and to enjoy your work. There is not much point in treating others when you have a negative, impatient, bored, or inattentive attitude. It will show in your work; people will notice and lose confidence in you and the treatment. In fact, if you can strive to develop a relaxed, peaceful, and compassionate state of mind, then this will greatly assist the effectiveness of the treatment. You may think that this is impossible: How can a state of mind positively affect an apparently physical therapy? Well, you can look at this in different ways. If you went to see a therapist who had an impatient and condescending attitude, this would make you feel uncomfortable; but if you are in the company of people who are peaceful and caring, you naturally feel some benefit from their presence.

Many people also believe that the therapist is also acting as a channel for healing energy, and that reflexology can act as a kind of energetic gateway for the patient to receive this. Definitely some people have a natural ability to heal others simply through touch, and it is often those that are attracted to the healing professions that possess such latent healing potential.

To successfully channel such healing energy from wherever you believe it comes from, you need a peaceful and relaxed mind, a feeling of compassion or empathy for your patient, and a wish for him or her to receive whatever he or she needs without grasping at success or being worried about failure in this regard. If you believe in a particular religion, then faith is very important. You can always say silent prayers for your patient before each treatment and ask for guidance, blessings, and healing inspiration.

If you do not see regular cures, you should not be surprised, disappointed, or discouraged. You do not know what people really need in their lives. It is difficult to see the "big picture," and sometimes there is a lot to be gained from someone having to develop the inner resources to live with a challenging illness. If you can impart this information skillfully and at the right time, then you may be doing your client a greater favor than if you were to simply take away his or her illness or disability.

Number of Treatments

How long and how frequently you treat someone depends on how much treatment he or she needs and how much time you are prepared to give. Usually a full treatment once a week is more than adequate. You may do this for six to eight weeks, and then reduce it to every two weeks and then once a month until a complete cure is established, or until the patient is happy with the outcome and doesn't feel the need to continue. In more serious and long-term cases, once a week is still usually enough, but it is really up to the patient to decide how long he or she wishes to continue regular treatments. Occasionally when people are very ill, two gentle half-hour treatments per week are more pleasant, relaxing, and less demanding on the body's ability to expel the toxins that are being released. Also, overstimulating a body's healing system that is already overtaxed with a serious illness can cause more problems. The answer is "gently does it."

Some people may not need any follow-up treatments after the initial six or eight, and some people may just want to come for, perhaps, three treatments, as a seasonal detoxification and revitalizing treatment. So you are not only there to help treat and relieve ailments and disease, but to also act as a life-enhancing and revitalizing therapist.

You can usually tell after the first three or four treatments if the condition you are treating is going to respond favorably to reflexology. This may not always be the case, although there are few instances of this occurring. Some people may find other complementary therapies to be more appropriate for them. Of course, most complementary therapies are complementary! The patient could be using two or three therapies at the same time without adverse effects. Again, the only thing you need to be wary of is that the body needs time to recover from detoxification, and too much treatment can make the patient feel ill while detox is occurring. In this regard, the more severe the illness, the gentler and more patient you must be with the patient.

Detoxification

Occasionally a "cleansing" period of the body and mind may occur after the first few reflexology treatments. This detoxification might be especially true if the patient has a serious illness. The effects of detox might include:

- Short-term minor illness (i.e., cold, flu)
- Sweating
- Headaches
- Frequent urination
- Increased sleepiness
- Increased thirst
- Temporary loss or increase in appetite
- Other minor physical problems or emotional release (i.e., crying, laughing)

It is not necessary for us to mention this to the patient as it does not always happen, but it is useful for us to remember this for when it does. These symptoms are a positive sign that the patient's body is working well to heal itself and we can encourage the client by telling them this. Although it is not a definite sign that they will regain health, so as always be careful what you say. If symptoms of detox are persistent and severe, reduce the regularity of treatments, the length of treatment, or use a gentler touch on the feet. Again, encouraging the patient to drink plenty of clean water, perhaps even three or four pints a day, can also help.

Treating Children

You can treat children the same way as adults. However, unless they are very ill, their attention span and, hence, their ability to lie still for a full treatment may be limited. You can either give shorter, more frequent treatments or treat them when they are asleep or sitting in their parent's lap. Obviously if you do not know the child well, a parent or guardian must be present throughout the treatment. It's not surprising that children are usually more naturally understanding and intuitively wise to natural healing techniques; consequently this trust and openness often brings swifter results.

Encouraging Healing

There are some things you can suggest to patients to help their natural healing process. These guidelines are not essential and not everyone would find them helpful, so only suggest them to patients if you think they are appropriate.

- Eat a healthy, well-balanced diet, including lots of fresh fruit and vegetables
- Cut down on alcohol
- Cut down on smoking or stop altogether if you can
- Avoid caffeinated drinks; instead drink lots of mineral water or herbal teas
- Cut down on chocolate, sweets, and other refined foods

- Try to eat only fresh food products
- Consider a short-term water or juice fast, but only if the patient has experience with fasting
- Avoid confrontational or stressful situations; try to keep a peaceful, happy, and relaxed mind
- Spend some quiet time on your own in a peaceful place; go for walks in pleasant surroundings
- Meditate or pray for ten to twenty minutes each day, or simply spend this time in silence or reading a spiritual text
- Think positively; essentially try to approach life with a relaxed, positive, and open mind

The effects of following these simple guidelines can be quite dramatic. If you ask your patients to follow them all for at least seven days, or even better three weeks. They will see that these changes make a big difference in their state of well-being. These physical and mental benefits can really inspire patients to continue these guidelines for longer periods until they become regular habits. They are sowing the seeds for good health now and in the future.

Medical Advice

If you think a patient may have a serious, undetected physical problem, try not to alarm him or her but encourage the patient to see his or her own doctor, especially if the patient also feels something is not right. A patient should never be afraid to see another doctor for a second opinion about his or her current medical condition. If you are a professional complementary therapist, all of your clients who are seeking help for serious medical complaints should come to you after or while they are being treated by their own doctor.

Positive Fatigue

It is quite common for people to feel tired or sleepy for days after a treatment. This is a good sign that they are beginning to learn how to finally "open" and fully relax. Often the amount of stress we carry goes unnoticed as we move from one thing in life to another. The habit of stress and the layers of stress gradually accumulate in our system, both physically and mentally, to the extent that we never allow ourselves time to just "be" who we are. We can even build up and carry stress with us from one lifetime to another for many lifetimes. This accumulated stress acts as a barrier to healing, inner peace, and a sense of our timeless spirituality, to the extent that we forget our true nature as primarily spiritual beings. Practicing natural healing techniques, meditation, prayer, or deep relaxation is a way to gradually release stress, cleanse the body/mind, and re-introduce us to ourselves.

Learning to deeply relax, open our mind, and allow stress, often in the form of negative thought patterns, to arise from within and fall away can sometimes be unnerving. We often feel these aspects of our mind are part of our own sense of self or true identity. This process can sometimes leave us feeling a little naked and unsure. However, given time and a little positive experience, we will develop the confidence and wish to consciously seek and appreciate this inner path toward a more whole and healthy way of living and being.

Heal Thyself

You can only be an effective healer if you can "heal" yourself. On the surface it appears that reflexology is just a physical therapy, but it is much more than this. The client/therapist relationship is of paramount importance. Obviously, any patient would be put off by an overbearing, self-important, and "loud" therapist. These qualities would leave the patient in doubt about the abilities and effectiveness of the therapist. Conversely, if the reflexologist is quietly confident, kind, considerate, patient, and willing to listen, then this can immediately instill confidence and a certain amount of faith and encouragement in the patient.

As a therapist you need to be in a frame of mind that allows the patient to feel comfortable and at ease. You really need to be at a place in your own mental and spiritual evolution where you have developed certain qualities that allow you to be a catalyst for healing. This may sound a little mystical, but it is a truth. If you are shallow, materialistic, self-centered, and in it for the money, praise, or recognition from others, then you really have nothing to give.

So how do you develop the special qualities that will transform you into an effective therapist? You really have to work this out for yourself, however, the first step is simply to develop the wish to be such a person, and much of the rest is simply learning from life experiences and interpreting them with wisdom. Some people find that following a recognized path of spiritual and personal growth to be very helpful.

Dealing with and Healing Patients

In everyday life we meet some people that we feel uncomfortable with and some people that we just don't like. If you are faced with this situation with a reflexology client, not liking the patient will not affect the quality of the treatment, but it will obviously affect the quality of the client/therapist relationship. In these situations, try to develop a warm and friendly professional relationship equally with all of your patients, without being particularly attached to some or adverse to others. Another strategy is to use the situation to discover more about yourself: Why do I not like this person? What is this situation telling me about myself?

Often the people and situations that we find difficult to deal with are reflections of some part of our own mind that we do not fully "own" or understand, like a missing piece of the puzzle. This also applies to situations or people we are deeply attached to or depend on for our happiness and peace of mind. Most relationships are tainted with aspects of need or aversion.

Often we need the approval or simply the presence of others to feel secure, happy, and whole, and it easy to think of many things we dislike or disapprove of in others. We don't have to be completely self-sufficient and separate, or completely reliant on others for our well-being—there is a middle way. We can learn to give and receive without needing others to feel whole or pushing others away to feel "free." This way of living leads to meaningful relationships and a sense of personal freedom. This feeling of equanimity is also a good attribute to develop and apply to all areas of our lives. If we try to cultivate a balanced, warm, and friendly attitude toward everyone we meet, all of our relationships will be naturally harmonious.

On the whole, given the right conditions, everyone has the natural ability to heal himself or herself. In some ways, being a reflexologist gives us the ability to provide these healing conditions, when others cannot initially help themselves. The less we interfere with this process the better. Too much good-intentioned advice can confuse people who may be already trying to deal with a difficult illness and changes in their life. We don't always know what is best for others. Often we want to give what others do not need, and trying to provide answers for others can lessen their ability to resolve their own issues. The "good" healer, to some extent, steps back from being a "solver of problems" and becomes more of an enabler, or simply, a healing witness. This allows people to draw through the healer, and from within themselves, what they actually need to help them overcome or transform their own situation either physically, mentally, or emotionally. This "sustainable healing" allows people to develop the qualities that either consciously or subconsciously they need to help themselves. It also provides them with the skills they may need to deal with similar problems in the future. This can be a slow process at first, but gradually healing the inner problems lays the foundation for a deep and lasting overall healing that is more than worth a little extra time and effort.

There is usually a strong connection between the problems people bring to you as a healer and your own issues; so if you seem to be attracting people with similar problems, this is an indication that you may need to move forward in those areas as well. You cannot expect other people to change for the better if you are not prepared to be honest about and challenge your own shortcomings. You do not have to be perfect, just prepared to learn more about yourself.

You should never feel pride about being a healer or act in a superior way; this can be a real barrier to your own healing and to improving your own healing abilities. If you try to be honest about your weaknesses, without being hard on yourself, and if you are able to share your problems and ask for help when you need it, then your own ability to heal yourself and others will continue.

As mentioned before, some people may not always get what they want from a reflexology treatment or what you would like them to receive. The cause of all illness has its root in the mind and therein also lies the cure of all illness. If the mind is not ready or willing to change on an obvious or subtle level, the illness will not be cured, or there may only achieve temporary relief. It appears that everyone has the wish to be healthy, however, very few people know themselves well enough to recognize that their illness is an expression of some part of their mind that does not wish to be healthy or that does not know how to be well. We can reteach ourselves to be well if we are willing to be patient and look within for the answers and not hand over the responsibility for our health to others.

Healing works on all levels but principally on a mental and emotional level first, so don't be surprised if a physical condition does not disappear overnight. Good reflexology works to achieve long-term improvements by helping the patient address, heal, and release the issues that initially caused the problem and this may happen obviously or in a very subtle way. Sometimes just learning to accept and live with a major illness is all you can help people achieve, depending on the severity and duration of the problem. You should never regard this as failure. If the patient's quality of life has improved only a little, you should be pleased with this progress.

Motivation and Dedication

There are two simple things you can do to make your healing actions more powerful and meaningful. If you are preparing to practice reflexology on yourself or others, you can begin with a short prayer, affirmation, or mental intention, finishing with a brief dedication.

Intention is everything! Your intention is what creates your karma. Although this is explained in more detail later, karma is everything you do, say, and think. Every action of body, speech, and mind creates a potential in the mind for a corresponding physical, verbal, or mental reaction in the future. It also creates the habit or tendency for you to repeat such actions in the future—an increased wish or compulsion to keep performing similar negative actions. If you perform negative actions, you can expect negative reactions sooner or later. Also, if you generally have a negative approach to life, you are more likely to create the conditions that attract problems and difficult circumstances. Likewise the positive energy you create by developing, patience, kindness, or by giving a reflexology treatment will return to you as a very positive experience in one form or another.

If you set a positive mental intention before performing any type of healing action, including reflexology, or indeed any form of giving or beneficial action, then this will greatly increase the power of your karma. If this intention is wise and heartfelt, the consequences of your actions can benefit countless living beings, although you cannot directly see this incredible result. Basically, if your motivation is to benefit others rather than yourself, then this will create powerful and positive karma.

To set an intention, you just need to sit quietly for a few minutes, calm the mind, and think of those people you would like to benefit. Then you can simply think or pray:

*Through the force of these healing actions may
(name the people you are thinking of) find
lasting happiness and good health.*

Or, even more powerfully:

*May every living being benefit from these
healing actions for their greatest good.*

Once you have finished the treatment, you can
dedicate your positive actions or good karma. Dedication is similar to intention. If you consciously dedicate,
or direct, this positive energy for a specific purpose,
this can be a very powerful way of manifesting your
intentions, achieving your goals, and accelerating your
spiritual or personal growth. Whenever you create positive energy by helping others in any way or by consciously developing positive states of mind, you can
dedicate this energy.

Choosing a purpose or direction for dedication is
similar to creating an intention. If you can choose a
purpose that will benefit many people, then this wish
will be fulfilled more easily than a purely selfish purpose. To dedicate after any positive action, simply
think or pray:

*May this positive energy be fully dedicated for
the greatest good of all living beings.*

Or:

*May every living being benefit from this
positive energy.*

Perhaps the greatest goals you could wish for are:

> *Through the force of this positive energy may*
> *every living being be released from suffering*
> *and may we all find true lasting happiness*
> *swiftly and easily.*

And/or:

> *Through the force of these positive actions may*
> *my wisdom and compassion continually*
> *increase for the benefit of others.*

Dedicating the positive energy created by your actions only takes a short time, but this small gesture is a very special practice. You can easily waste or destroy the potential of previous positive actions, or good karma, simply by developing negative states of mind like anger, guilt, or jealousy. Sincere and heartfelt dedication is like "banking" or protecting the potential of your positive actions for your own and other's future benefit. In this way, the potential of your good thoughts, words, and deeds can only increase and will produce excellent results for yourself and everyone in the future.

Not many people practice reflexology for the money. If you want to dedicate your life to the accumulation of material wealth, then reflexology is probably not the path for you. However, if you are interested in using your time to help cure and relieve illness, and you want to practice a therapy that is powerful, gentle, intimate, yet noninvasive, then reflexology might be your vocation. Certainly, you will gain great personal satisfaction from seeing the pleasure and peace others derive from your healing actions—paid or unpaid. If you have a genuine concern for the welfare of others, you will be a good reflexologist.

7

Case Studies

In a book like this, it is important to share with the reader the ideas and experiences of other professionals working in this field of complementary therapy. This chapter gives a range of stories, advice, interesting articles, and research results of the effectiveness of reflexology. It is hoped that the reader will gain a little insight into the types of people that practice reflexology and an appreciation of what a wonderfully healing and helping therapy it can be.

How I Became a Reflexologist

My interest in reflexology was aroused by my daughter Kiri. Kiri was born deaf, and after completing her formal education, she decided to train as a beauty therapist. During her third year of training, Kiri was given the opportunity to add certain options. Initially she had wanted to learn reflexology but found the course to be full, and so she opted for aromatherapy instead.

When finally qualified, Kiri started work and was asked by one employer if she would consider undertaking a reflexology course. Kiri agreed to this and began to search for a course. She found one at the local college that offered a diploma in reflexology. Kiri decided that this course would suit her needs, and so she and I went to meet with a tutor.

Being deaf, Kiri needed the services of a note-taker to help her understand the theory sessions. The services of a note-taker can prove very expensive, and so I asked if I could act as her note-taker. The tutor suggested that I enroll in the course myself. This would enable me to gain a professional qualification and also help Kiri at the same time.

Upon completing the course and passing the examination, I felt extremely proud to have obtained my diploma. However, this was only the beginning. Since then, I have gone on to do another course that has enabled me to become a full member of the Association of Reflexologists (MAR).

Working as a reflexologist has given me new confidence, a greater understanding of people, and has given me many opportunities to work and meet with people I otherwise would never have met. It has also given me the friendship of several wonderfully caring people.

Ironically, Kiri has never used reflexology since completing the course. She has chosen to concentrate solely on beauty therapy and is extremely good at her job, with a many happy and satisfied clients.

For me, reflexology has become a fascinating art and science, and something I do not think I will ever stop learning about. So I would like to thank my wonderful daughter without whom I would never have discovered such an interesting and beneficial therapy. Thank you, Kiri!

Maureen Warwick, MAR

Thirty-five Pairs of Feet in a Week

I have just had my busiest week ever, giving thirty-five reflexology treatments, including two days of corporate reflexology. This is one of the biggest achievements of my life as only eighteen months ago I was still working as a consultant, and eighteen months before that I was unable to get out of bed due to postviral syndrome (chronic fatigue syndrome). At age twenty-four, I knew there must be more to life, and such an illness makes you realize what is really important. My job was seriously affecting my health and reflexology helped me recover, so it seemed it was a natural path to follow. Hence, I set about the difficult task of changing my career and life to one that is now infinitely more fulfilling.

It has not been an easy journey, and I am sure there are more problems (or, should I say, opportunities) to come. I have had to make some scary decisions to get to this point, not the least of which was actually resigning from my high-powered, well-paid consulting job, with no job to go to.

In the early days of practice, I reluctantly supplemented my income by holding business awareness courses in large corporations on a contract basis. It was only when I finally (and scarily!) let go of this last thread of my old life that my reflexology practice truly took off. I knew what a drain on my energy the training had been, but fear had stopped me letting go earlier.

I started off my practice in a state-registered chiropodist's facility on a commission basis. This gave me a large existing client base to tap into but no fixed costs to pay out every week—perfect! I now work two full days a week there, and it is lovely to get out of the house and still feel part of something, too.

Alongside this I built up my home practice in Chester by renting booths at natural health exhibitions, open evenings at a local gym, and a distributing a few leaflets and posters. A professional, eye-catching exhibition stand is vital and a Relaxator chair is always a hit!

Without a doubt I have had some luck—if there is such a thing—such as the gentleman whose feet I did at an exhibition. When I had finished, he stood up and said, "I think you had better come and do my staff." Hence, my first corporate client!

I now average twenty to twenty-five pairs of feet a week, mostly hour-long treatments. I have tried to develop a unique, or at least different, offering to my clients. Over the eighteen months since I received my qualifications, I have attended several postgraduate workshops (including vitality reflexology) to extend my "toolbox" of techniques, enabling me to adapt each treatment to each client each time they come. In fact, I was so inspired by the courses I attended at the Association of Reflexologists Summer School in Chester last year that I decided to become involved in organizing this year's event.

I also believe customer feedback is vital, and I frequently send out questionnaires. They can be relatively expensive but have a number of uses. They can prompt clients to reflect and recognize benefits gained; be a real confidence booster for you; help highlight any areas of improvement; help encourage clients to come back (as a gentle reminder); provide you with some good quotes for marketing material. You won't, of course, get them all back, but I have found they do more than pay for themselves overall.

While this tale is sounding too good to be true, I have made mistakes, had major confidence crises (although now I only have the odd minor one), and followed paths that have not been worthwhile either financially, time-wise, or just too restricting. I believe this is all part of the learning process. It is as important to find out what you don't want to do as it is to find out what you do! Forget what everyone else is doing and search for what suits you—whether that is thirty-five pairs of feet in three different locations or three home visits a week, the important thing is that you and your clients are happy!

The other day I thought how odd my job must seem to many people, but I also realized that I was at work and was not wishing I was somewhere else—a good sign that I have found what I want to do. While there is no substitute for hard work in building up a practice, I also know I have received a lot of support: Adele; everyone at the chiropody practice; Nick (my incredibly patient husband); Simon Duncan (my tutor and "sounding board"); friends and fellow reflexologists; and, of course, my clients, without whom there would be no practice!

Whatever stage you are at, I wish you all luck and hope that you find reflexology as fulfilling to receive and give as I do!

Kate Scarborough, MAR

A Common Ailment Cured by Reflexology

Mr. A. arrived for his reflexology session complaining of severe headaches. It transpired that he had suffered whiplash about five years earlier and had suffered soft tissue damage to his neck. He was in pain, lied awake at night, and generally was miserable. He took a wide range of strong painkillers on a regular basis and did not know where to turn.

During consultation, we covered his dietary habits. He was very much a convenience-food man. As he put it, his parents were in favor of the "greasy spoon"-type breakfasts, and that is how he had been brought up. However, he wanted to change and to follow a healthy diet, even though his family thought it odd. The reflexology sessions gave him a chance to discuss healthy options to his lifestyle; perhaps he did not have the chance to do this elsewhere. Consequently, he would often solve his own questions: "I could take an apple and a banana to work instead of a snack pot!"

During the initial consultation, he revealed he only had a bowel movement every five days—sometimes longer! During treatment, the large intestine reflex was found to be hard, with a callus at the rectum reflex point. His neck and shoulder reflexes were gritty, and he felt a lot of tension release when these were worked on. After his first session he arrived home and immediately needed use the bathroom, and did so again later that evening. He said he felt "lighter." He came regularly for his weekly sessions, and within a short space of time, he was having bowel movements every two days, especially soon after treatment. His headaches changed almost immediately from continuous to rarely. Motivated by the dramatic improvement, he changed to a whole-grain cereal breakfast, started drinking more water, and took fruit as a snack to work. He continues his reflexology to this day and does not suffer from headaches. He totally relaxes when he comes, and says he has regained control of his life.

Reflexology had such an immediate effect on his constipation that he was quite amazed. He has since tried other complementary therapies but finds reflexology to be such a physical benefit as well as a relaxing one that he goes nowhere else.

Caroline Killalea, MAR

A Case Study

This case study was carried out in 1997 while I was training in reflexology.

Ms. C. is a twenty-four-year-old female with special educational needs. She currently attends a life skills class at a local college. As I have no communication with Ms. C.'s family, I have been unable to obtain a full medical history. However Ms. C. does not smoke or consume alcohol. She appears extremely nervous and insecure, is inclined to be hyperactive at times, and suffers from severe psoriasis, which covers her entire body. When I first met Ms. C., she was extremely hostile toward me; she wanted to hit me and said that she hated me. Eventually her caregiver persuaded her to remove her shoes and socks and lie on the treatment couch. Upon examination of her feet, it appeared that she might be mutilating herself. There were several deep slashes on her feet as well as many patches of psoriasis. The areas most severely affected were the thyroid, lungs, bronchial, ears and eyes, and shoulder reflexes.

During the first treatment, I was only able to perform very gentle relaxation movements to the feet because of the lacerations and psoriasis. It was really a case of sitting there and gently holding her feet. Gradually Ms. C. began to relax and then started to cry. At one point she became almost hysterical, crying and sobbing. She said that she was very frightened at the thought of leaving the college environment, where she felt safe, and going to a new day center later in the year.

At the end of the first treatment, Ms. C. was much more relaxed and had accepted me as "her friend." She asked to come back for another treatment.

Subsequent treatments showed a marked improvement in the psoriasis and lacerations to her feet. At the fourth treatment, all the lesions had healed and new, healthy skin growth was clearly visible. Ms. C. is now much calmer and has a more positive outlook regarding her future. She is also becoming more confident and more communicative with me. If I meet her around the college, she will now rush over to hug me and tells people, "This is my friend. She does my feet." Ms. C.'s mother has been so impressed with the improvement in her daughter's skin that she called to say, "I have never seen her skin look so good."

At the end of six treatments, Ms. C.'s feet and legs were completely clear of psoriasis. Her tutors had commented that she was much calmer and quieter in class, was more relaxed, and now looked forward to going to the new day center.

Initially, Ms. C. would only attend treatment if her caregiver sat with her. However, for the final treatment, Ms. C. allowed me to collect her from her class and bring her to the treatment room where she has happily received treatment without the caregiver in attendance.

I was so impressed with the difference that reflexology made to Ms. C. that I offered to continue to treat her at home. Unfortunately, this offer was refused by Ms. C's mother who is agoraphobic and allows no one, apart from close family, to enter the home. Upon visiting the college some months later, I saw Ms. C. I was distressed to find that she had reverted to being hyper-active again and that her psoriasis had come back with a vengeance. Ms. C. was delighted to see me and asked me to "do my feet please." Sadly my offer to treat Ms. C. is still rejected by her mother.

Reflexology definitely helped Ms. C. to become relaxed, and this in turn helped her psoriasis heal. This was evident upon seeing her again following a period when she was not being treated.

Maureen Warwick, MAR

Reflexology and Her Supporting Aspects

Let us just presume that more than 1,000 reflexology charts exist worldwide and that these reflexology charts are a guide for many thousands of practicing reflexologists. Imagine also that these reflexologists use different ways of treatment, like working with oil, talcum powder, wooden sticks or metal objects, a flat thumb, or with knuckles. One could say there are thousands of different ways of expressing foot reflexology. And they all really work. So could there be another important factor, which is the red thread running through all these various methods of treatment?

The answer is "yes!" It is my positive conviction that you, the reflexologist, are the "supporting and connecting factor." It is not only the technical perform-ance that you give but also the passion and love that is felt by the patient during the treatment, often uncon-sciously.

Of course, the clients who seek your help are often in pain, grief, or sorrow, and it is your attention, respect, and consolation that helps them to relax in body and mind. Furthermore, there is the listening factor. You are able to listen to your client for more than three-quarters of an hour, and this also has great value, as listening has become a lost art in this part of the world.

When client and therapist are "on the same frequency," there can become a collective consciousness, in which the client is lifted up and can see intuitively the cause of his or her problem. Or, in another sense, the therapist functions as a mirror (reflex!), and the client recognizes the cause of his illness and then has the possibility to work on that.

So let us be aware of the fact that the "supporting aspect" in foot reflexology is a very important factor—and once more, that factor is you. You are the motivated, caring, passionate, loving person behind reflexology, because in reality that is in fact what you are—passion and love.

Henk Homberg
founder and former chairman,
Association of European Reflexologists

Bach Flower Remedies and Reflexology

I have been practicing reflexology since 1996 and have been familiar with the Bach Flower Remedies since 1981, when I first experienced their powerful influence. I had forgotten how magical they were until Maxine

Rawlings gave our local group of reflexologists a talk on the Bach Flower Remedies. I was captured by her enthusiasm and instantly wanted to learn more. A group of us persuaded her to start an evening class here in Brighton. We did a weekly course of two hours for ten weeks and learned a great deal from Maxine. We also had a lot of fun!

Kitty McCormick, a fellow reflexologist, and I took our training a little further by attending the Bach Flower Remedy Practitioner's Course at the Bach Flower Remedy Centre in Oxfordshire. It was here that Dr. Bach lived and worked, preparing his remedies using the flowers from the surrounding countryside. For me it was very special as I come from this part of country, and it brought back many memories. I was also fascinated by the idea that Dr. Bach's little cottage, in its beautiful setting and with its magic, was a stone's throw from where I grew up! As a child I had no idea that it even existed.

Since my training, I have used the flower remedies alongside reflexology with outstanding results. I feel that the remedies work extremely well with reflexology to enhance healing, well-being, and peace of mind. An example of this is a client who came regularly for foot reflexology. She was experiencing a recurring nightmare, which had plagued her for years. I suggested some flower remedies, and this improved her general well being, but the dream still continued. Suddenly it struck me that the Pine remedy would be the answer. Pine is the remedy for guilty feelings. The client took the remedy eighteen months ago and has not had the dream since.

This same remedy produced a surprising reaction in a male client. After two weeks of taking Pine, he came back saying, "What did you put in that bottle?" I replied, "Why?" "Well," he said, "I have become more amorous!" I must admit I was a bit taken aback, but these are powerful little drops!

The thirty-eight Bach Flower Remedies are not only a powerful tool, but have also helped me to understand and recognize states of mind in myself, in my clients, and those around me. Each remedy has the qualities of a specific state of mind. These states of mind are usually recognized by the negative qualities. I feel my "toolkit" is enormously enhanced by my rediscovery and use of the Bach Flower Remedies.

These remedies are essentially a vibrational healing therapy and are used by matching the vibration of the person to the vibration of the remedy, in much the same way as in homeopathy. The positive aspects of the person are enhanced, allowing the negative aspects to drop away. For example, Impatiens, the remedy for impatience, would be used for a negative state of impatience, thus bringing about patience. Olive would be used for exhaustion, bringing about a feeling of restfulness. White Chestnut would be used for recurring thoughts, resulting in a more peaceful mind.

I would recommend any reflexologist to take an interest in the remedies. Take the time to learn the qualities of each one, and use them when it feels appropriate. If you are interested in the Bach Flower

Remedies, go and learn about them and experiment. They are great fun and fascinating—a natural resource not to be missed!

Ella Preece, MAR

How Reflexology Helped Me to Have an Easier Labor

Like most mothers, particularly first-time moms, I was very anxious about giving birth. I had a positive attitude and decided I didn't want pain relief. I didn't want pethidine, an epidural, a cesarean, or an episiotomy unless absolutely necessary.

I am qualified in aromatherapy and reflexology and have a lot of faith in them, particularly reflexology. During my pregnancy I attended a maternity reflexology course, which was excellent. It taught me that reflexology can reduce labor time by up to half, is totally safe to use throughout pregnancy, and has many benefits. I already had a couple of treatments and met a mobile reflexologist at the course who treated me weekly from when I was twenty weeks along. It relieved my backache and helped me to sleep; I was very calm and relaxed. I also took raspberry leaf tea capsules at thirty-six weeks and made an oil containing the essential oils of lavender and jasmine to help the backache and help the uterus to contract. This can be used in the bath and in massage on the back and abdomen. It can also be used during labor.

Our baby was due on November 19, 2000. On November 14, I started getting twinges at about 6 A.M.

I went into the hospital at 10 A.M. when my contractions were coming every four minutes. I was examined at 11:15 A.M. and was only 2 centimeters dilated. At 1 P.M. my contractions were every two minutes and very strong. I got into the birthing pool at around 1:30 P.M. but was only in there for about twenty minutes as I couldn't get comfortable. My contractions were now every minute and my water broke at 2:30 P.M. (It was quite a gush and my two birthing partners and myself had very wet feet!) I was examined again and was now 10 centimeters dilated. Using gas and air, Olivia was born at 2:59 P.M. with no pushing—she just came out.

I believe that I had a very easy labor and birth. I am not saying it wasn't painful—because it was—but it was not as bad as I thought it would be, and the second I saw Olivia, I fell in love with her.

I strongly believe that being calm and relaxed, along with a positive attitude and the complementary therapies that I used, helped me to have the easy and quick labor that I wanted. I thoroughly recommend that every pregnant woman has reflexology, if possible, as the benefits are very rewarding.

Our baby is calm and content, and I believe that me having reflexology has made her this way. I am now practicing it on her, which she seems to enjoy, and have recommended it to some friends whose babies have suffered with colic and constipation; they, too, have had positive results.

Lisa Holyland

The Emotional Benefits of Reflexology

Much can be said of the benefits that complementary therapies, including reflexology, can have for the mind, body, and spirit. Indeed, people often report improvements in physical conditions ranging from backaches and stress to fertility problems, skin complaints, and asthma. But in my experience, the most marked and extensive improvements are continually found in the emotional state of the client. When a client comes for a treatment, there is usually at least a little disquiet in his or her mind, and in various cases I've treated, the client has been severely emotionally unstable. Yet when the client gets up to leave, he or she will, in almost all cases, say that he or she "feels" much better and usually report an improvement in his or her moods between treatments. After a number of treatments, it has been possible to see very clearly, especially in more severe cases of emotional upset, that the client is finding an inner solace and strength that had previously been lost.

This is particularly encouraging in cases where chronic emotional problems are present, as it gives the client hope and faith that there are treatment options where other conventional methods may have failed. I certainly found this to be the case when working last year at a charity for sufferers of anxiety disorders. Many of the people I treated were relieved to find that reflexology soothed them in ways that counseling and drugs had been unable to. They rediscovered a little peace of mind they had almost forgotten existed! In my opinion, reflexology has its greatest potential here.

Certainly, as a preventative therapy, a happy, relaxed mind goes a long way to maintaining a healthy, relaxed body. This, in turn, leads to an efficient immune system and a thorough elimination of toxins. Also, in cases where a physical condition is present, that can also be improved; the client is in a positive and relaxed state of mind because it is resting, free of fears and worries, so that the body heals.

It's important to remember, however, that the road to recovery is not always a straight one. On occasions a strong and sometimes unpleasant reaction follows a treatment. This is particularly the case when there is a condition caused by a hormonal imbalance. For example, in a case such as polycystic ovary syndrome, a client may experience a day or two of feeling tearful, emotional, unstable, or aggressive. This is, of course, a healing reaction, and the client always comes to a more balanced, improved point following this reaction. But it is important to inform clients that this is a common reaction and part of the healing process, and that it will pass. They must be sure that they are suitably supported and happy to embark on this road to recovery.

You may find it helpful if you can explain to clients why they might have a reaction like this. It is also beneficial to explain why reflexology ultimately makes them feel better.

So what is it in a reflexology treatment that causes these changes in emotion?

The technique itself causes changes to the circulation and, therefore, the physiological state of the client. There are many views on how exactly this takes place and the consequent effects, but I believe that this is only a part of the powerful impact reflexology has on the emotional state. I believe the other significant influence of change comes from the treatment process as a whole. In other words, it is what we can give and receive as humans to one another that can alter, to an impressive degree, our emotional status. We all know that being nice to people makes them feel good, but it is the following conditions that take clients into a realm of healing that conventional treatment cannot:

The importance of touch: This is a heavily studied area in many fields, and there is evidence to show that the human body responds to the effect of a caring, nurturing touch in very positive ways.

The importance of being listened to: Although reflexologists are not counselors, the time spent discussing a client's case history is important. Because the process is holistic, the client feels that he or she is being considered as a whole and that nothing is being dismissed or treated as inappropriate.

Time to allow themselves a treat: Many people, especially those with emotional problems, find it hard to allow themselves treats, but the gentle nature of reflexology quiets those beliefs and draws the client to a feeling of worthiness.

Positive exchange of energy: So often in life when we interact with one another, we are battling for energy. We do this without realizing how draining and negative it is. However, during a treatment, the therapist is focused on the well-being of the client and is offering kindness and support unconditionally. This is positively energizing for the client and also the therapist.

Opportunity to take control and heal themselves: Our minds and bodies often become depressed and ill due to feelings of fear, stress, and helplessness. Showing clients that they and their bodies have the ability to heal naturally from within empowers them and encourages them to take control of their well-being with a respect for their bodies.

Deeper relaxation: Anyone who has had reflexology treatments will comment on the profound sensation of relaxation during and after a treatment. The level of relaxation is similar to that achieved during meditation. This is truly the wonder of reflexology. The benefits of this balance and peace on an individual's emotional state are obvious.

Of course, these are only the views of one reflexologist. You may have many an inspiring and interesting time as a therapist or client testing out the ideas here and coming up with some of your own. I don't claim to be a scientist nor should I, but I do claim to believe that reflexology has huge potential as a treatment option for people suffering from long-term emotional problems (not to be confused with psychological disorders) and have experienced many case studies to prove to this effect. If you haven't tried reflexology yet, maybe now is the time to find out what all the fuss is about. If you find it difficult to afford a treatment, try offering yourself as a case study to a student of reflexology at one of the schools. Alternatively, you could get more books from the library and try some self-treatment reflexology. Enjoy!

S. J. B. Barnett, MAR

A Case Study

Charlotte is thirteen years old, eats a healthy diet, consisting of two portions of vegetables every day. Her mother loves cooking, so most of the food is fresh and homemade. Charlotte also loves sports. But due to the extreme pain her menstrual periods bring, she has taken too much time off of school so that now her schoolwork is suffering.

Her periods started when she was twelve. On the first day, the pain was so bad that her doctor thought that she had appendicitis. Her doctor also suggested that she "has big ovaries," which he said accounted for the pain and heavy blood loss. The period lasted fourteen days, and during that time she was in pain and could not go to school, as the pain grew worse when she walked.

The pain keeps her awake at night, so she is tired most of the time. Her periods generally last for twelve to fourteen days. Then when she turned thirteen, the period started lasting longer, anywhere up to seventeen days, with only nine days with no period. The pain was extreme, forcing her to take 600 milligrams of ibuprofen every five hours. She found she could not wait the normal six hours as the pain was too severe.

She also has had warts and verucas since the age of ten and made numerous visits to consultants within the National Health Service and the private sector. Having tried to burn them out, dig them out, and cut them out, and used creams, lotions, and whatever else the doctor gave her to apply only made them very sore and come back with a vengeance and spread further. The warts, quite large and cauliflower in shape, are on her fingers and thumbs, eyelids, and the tops of her legs and feet. Most of the warts on the hands and feet are about the size of a small fingernail. Verucas covers a large area of the soles of her feet, which hurt when she walks. She also suffers from seasonal sinus problems. She does not sleep very well and is quite restless during the night. Apart from her medical ailments, she is otherwise healthy and tries to lead an active life. Following are my clinical notes:

> **First treatment (March 15, 2000):** She was very nervous. Her feet were clammy, with a strong odor. The feet were pink and healthy looking with no hard skin. I started with the pituitary area and she started shaking from head to foot. She described it as a tidal wave traveling from her head downward. I covered her up with a towel, as she was distressed. On the right foot, the pituitary, hypothalamus, pineal, all sinus areas, adrenals, and all the reproductive areas were very painful. The trembling lasted right through to the end of

the treatment, but started to subside when I began the warm-down foot massage. By the time I had finished her entire treatment, she had stopped shaking. She was quite tearful afterward, but very positive.

Second treatment (March 22, 2000): The day after her first treatment she felt very tired, which lasted until Saturday, after which she felt fine. I was very pleased to be told that her period had only lasted eight days this time with hardly any pain, which I thought might be just coincidence, but Charlotte was pleased. Both feet were painful in the same areas, but there was no shaking this time. I noticed that the verucas were less protruding this time, and that she was generally more relaxed and more trusting this time around.

Third treatment (March 29, 2000): Charlotte felt very tired after the last treatment, which only lasted until the next day. Her sleep has improved and no sign of her period yet, but she had pain in her reproductive area on Sunday. She had very sore eyes, which looked like conjunctivitis. The wart on her big toe had shrunk. All reproductive reflex areas were sore as were the sinus and chest areas. Generally a good, positive treatment.

Fourth treatment: (April 3, 2000): Charlotte's period started on March 31, with no pain, and lasted one day. Then the pain was very bad for three days without period. She felt very tired after the last treatment. She saw her doctor who confirmed conjunctivitis and gave her antibiotic drops. The wart on her big toe looked smaller. She is more relaxed as treatment continues and I am pleased period is altering. All toe reflexes "crunchy" around sinus area, pituitary, and hypothalamus, and they hurt a lot during the treatment on both feet. She is now sleeping and dreaming deeply. Warts and verucas seem to be less obvious. On her hands they are sore but smaller and slightly bleeding, and the verucas are turning black on soles of feet. During the treatment, Charlotte relaxed and fell asleep.

Fifth treatment (April 12, 2000): April 11 brought period for one day. She feels sick and full of wind today, and says she feels like she is getting a cold. Wart on right big toe has reduced so much and is now hardly visible. Verucas on feet have all gone black. Reflexes for sinus and neck hurt, also pituitary and facial area, but then she told me about her bad toothache. Bowel reflex very "bubbly." On her left foot sinus area, head, and spinal lumbar area, painful. Very tired after treatment.

Sixth treatment (April 19, 2000): Still has excessive wind but not as bad; toothache still there but not as bad. Period cycle has changed drastically; sleeping much better but nails have started to crack. On the right foot, her womb reflex was very "crunchy" and felt odd; also all sinus area sore. Left foot: pituitary and two small toes "crunchy," and shoulder reflex sore. Throat area feels sore. Warts on hands almost gone, just red marks now. Verucas on feet are still black in the center. Verucas on big toe has gone. Hooray! She felt tired but happy.

Seventh treatment (April 26, 2000): Period lasts three days, no pain this time, but pain after treatment had finished, like a cramp. She has a throat infection and is on antibiotics, so I am only working reproductive area this week. Good treatment.

Eighth treatment (May 3, 2000): Throat infection Wednesday through Friday. She has been feeling quite poorly. Had full treatment but she felt very tired. Most reflex areas hurt, probably due to virus; sent her back to doctor.

Ninth treatment (May 17, 2000): Warts and verucas almost gone, only black centers on soles of feet, warts on hands and fingers have left blemishes (red), and warts on thighs and eyelids have gone without a trace. During last period, she hardly had any pain, and she really enjoys treatment now. All sinus areas sore, chest tight, but she was very tired. Good treatment.

Tenth treatment (May 24, 2000): Marks on hands from warts have completely gone, and so have all the others; only thing left is black centers in the middle of the verucas on sole of left foot in fifth zone, although it is not raised or sore. Sciatic area very painful on foot and lower back. Period started on May 21 (Sunday) and stopped that evening; on Tuesday it came again and lasted until that evening—very odd. All sinus reflex areas "crunchy" as was throat area on both feet, womb reflex very spongy, and she felt quite sleepy. Good treatment.

As the reflex treatments have been so successful with Charlotte's problems, namely her warts and verucas, I decided to continued on with fortnightly intervals, as it has altered her period cycle but has not corrected it. She is very pleased with the way her reflex treatments have gone after so many years of putting up with these problems.

I will be putting pen to paper in the next couple of days informing her doctor of the success with the warts and verucas, as I would like to think that this information would be of great help to future problems; and you never know, doctors might just start to refer cases like Charlotte's to reflexologists!

Patricia Eden, MAR

Freedom

Some years ago I wrote about freedom, but now, so many years later, freedom has a much greater meaning to me.

Having been a sounding board for the many people who have crossed my path, great value has been added to the ideas I had about freedom. Freedom has its limitations and I will come back to this point later on.

Freedom is, in a way, close to one's inner self. The self, in essence, is outgoing—open to truth, light, and love—but is often hindered by the many burdens we carry through life. I like to call it our rucksack filled with all the undigested emotions and unresolved actions or mistakes committed in the past.

We are entering a new earth period, and as we follow our chosen path through life, we can, by way of a complicated system of crossing over into another vibration, receive enlightenment, help, and fresh choices. This change of consciousness is necessary in order to receive insight into and understanding of these undigested emotions that still cling to us (part of the karma idea).

Acquiring freedom is an important link in our self-discovery. The various stages in reaching a state of self-liberation will become part of us, because we have dared to accept the opportunities we are offered (which often seem mysteriously accidental), and then cope with any trials and difficulties we meet along the way. By understanding the experiences, which are coupled to old emotions, we will be able to free ourselves again and again of the contents of the rucksack, which weigh us down and hold us back.

We will become lighter, not only because of the partly resolved karma, but mainly because we have become more transparent, and this in turn gives us access to other vibrations, vibrations that cannot be assimilated before we are ready to receive them.

If you are aware that this freedom is possible but are held back because you dare not open the door of your ego, you may find that "help" is being thrust upon you, for instance:

A. You would love to do something totally new, but after years and years of working within a strict routine, you are held up by the fear of unknown consequences. Then, out of the blue, you are fired from your job, and so, for whatever reason, you are free to fulfill your long-cherished wish. This is just one of the many ways you may receive help and the first glimpse of your chosen freedom.

B. You lose your partner either by accident, death, or separation and unexpectedly your life changes. This can also be seen as a form of freedom, which releases you from the emotional bonds which tied you to your partner.

C. You intuitively know that a moment has come in your life when you will have to make an important decision, but you deliberately choose to ignore this intuition. So perhaps you become ill or confined to bed for a long period so that you have the time to think about your life, and become curious about the purpose of this bedridden period. Then, after having received this insight, you understand the reason and are able to make that important decision.

Over the past years, I have witnessed the many and various forms of help that have been offered to people. Sometimes it seems too complicated to understand until, sometime in the future, we see the beauty and simplicity of that offered help. Again and again through are lives we are given the opportunity to reach some degree of freedom. In many cases, we do not actually see these possibilities as a part of our liberation, but rather worry about other aspects of that transformation.

Whenever and however it happens to you, if you let it happen, try to be open. Accept the offered adventure that was meant for you and for you only. Make it part of yourself and again your spirit will grow in freedom.

Remember things are not the way you think they are, but the way you feel them to be! So now and then, be the clown, be funny, laugh from the bottom of your belly, or say "no" for once. In fact, be like Jonathan Livingstone Seagull (book/film) and deny worldly obligations and expectations.

Do you hate birthdays? Then visit your friend some other day when you will have the opportunity for a real conversation with the person you love (on a heart-to-heart level), instead of having to chat for a whole evening about dull-headed subjects in a smoky room or hall. In fact, there are no obligations—don't let them be forced upon you. You are the one who decides! Feel free to be free!

Henk Homberg
Association of European Reflexologists

Reflections on Reflexology

It all began with my chronic back pain problem, which had been present since the birth of my third child many years before. On returning to work as a staff nurse in the National Health Service, I needed to sort things out. I had tried all the conventional things like doctors, physiotherapists, sugar injections, osteopaths, and even spinal injections. These worked only temporarily. Then, the padre who blessed our marriage told me how his seemingly "incurable" shoulder pain had been cured in two sessions with a local reflexologist whom I shall call Lyndsey.

I duly made an appointment with hope in my heart. The first treatment felt good and so relaxing, but Lyndsey warned me that I might feel ill afterward. This proved to be an understatement! Later that day I seemed to be going down with a bad case of the flu. I rang Lyndsey, as she had requested, and she reassured me. Apparently there was so much tension present in my back that "letting go" was bound to cause large repercussions. In a couple of days I felt fine and my pain shifted. I had ten treatments, and Lyndsey taught me how to manage and reduce the tension that causes and surrounds muscle spasms.

This experience so impressed me that I was determined to find out as much as I could about reflexology, and a few years later I enrolled in a course to become a reflexologist. I joined seven other students and we had a fascinating year together, eventually all passing the examinations required. During this year we had to complete six case histories of ten treatments each.

My own treatments of the six clients produced some fascinating effects. One lady, very frail and ill with Parkinson's disease, completely relaxed at the end of each treatment, and her tremors almost ceased for about twenty minutes. The second client had hypertension, among numerous other problems. Over the weeks her blood pressure was lowered. Another interesting but puzzling effect was on a client who otherwise didn't seem to respond very well. From the moment I massaged her eye reflexes each week, her eyes watered uncontrollably until the end of the session. However, the most rewarding consequence was to a client who had recently had a baby by in-vitro fertilization after years of infertility. She has recently telephoned to say she is pregnant again, this time by natural means, and is totally amazed and overjoyed. Although this happened some months after she finished her treatment, I like to think maybe reflexology had something to do with it.

With regard to learning reflexology, in spite of my medical training, I found the course examinations quite exacting mentally and physically. Everyone involved, including the teachers and examiners, were really helpful and put us at ease to help us succeed. I have now been qualified nearly a year and look forward to future years of helping people and hopefully enhancing my skills and knowledge.

Rita G. Cox, MAR

Low Thyroid Function—
The Undiagnosed Epidemic

In twelve years of reflexology practice I have come across many people with illnesses that do not change or get better despite treatment by their doctor. Thyroid dysfunction, which is easily picked up on the feet by a competent reflexologist, is one of those illnesses.

I was one of those people. I knew from treating my own feet that my pituitary wasn't happy: the reflex in my big toe throbbed constantly, I felt exhausted, and my hair was falling out by the handful. I had gained over twenty pounds and couldn't lose it. I tried every diet going and nothing worked. I was freezing all of the time, even in warm weather, and I could have slept for Britain!

I felt very lucky that my doctor sent off for blood tests, and I was diagnosed with low thyroid function. My doctor sent me to my local endocrinologist and placed me on medication. My luck ran out right there at the hospital. I was told that because I wasn't losing any weight and my blood tests said I was well again, that I should go home and stop "pigging out" and cut down on the alcohol—as if that had to be the reason! As eating regularly has always been a problem, and I do like a glass of wine now and then, I am still no raging alcoholic. I knew the doctor was wrong, but I couldn't get anyone to listen.

Although reflexology helped for four years, I struggled with the weight gain, tiredness, and coldness until I discovered the Internet and found others like myself.

I found out that the thyroid function blood test used is inaccurate and that doctors, even consultants, misinterpret them and leave people (mostly women) feeling ill, unable to function, and living half of a life.

Through the Internet I found Mary Shomon's website and her top doctor's list. From there I discovered doctors in the UK who will treat sufferers like me properly and make us well. I'm now feeling great and raring to go. I am creating a database of doctors who will treat patients according to their symptoms, not their blood tests, and of hospitals who will test correctly, so that people will know where they can go to for help.

That is the reason I set up the Thyroid Support Association UK. Patients need a voice and information, so that not only can they understand their condition, but they can give their doctor information to enable them to have the courage to do what they became doctors for—make people well.

(*See appendix 4 for additional information on hypothyroidism.*)

Gina Wright, MAR

Author's note: There is a growing volume of research papers around the world showing the beneficial effects of reflexology on mental and physical health. The following summaries of two research projects by Peta Trousdell serve to highlight growing interest in the effects of reflexology on health and well-being. It is this kind of dedicated and well-informed work that is bringing conventional medicine and complementary medicine closer together.

Reflexology Meets Emotional Needs

(This is a summary of an article by Peta Trousdell appearing in the International Journal of Complementary Medicine, *November 1996. The article is detailed and extensive and so only a small section can be presented here.)*

The research was carried out between February and April 1996. Fifteen women who attended the Threshold Drop-in groups in Coldean, Brighton, and Hove, took part in the project over a period of eleven weeks. Each woman received reflexology treatments once a week for eight weeks, lasting thirty minutes. At each subsequent treatment, the reflexologists sought to establish with the women what sort of effects they felt the treatment had. Open-ended, semistructured individual interviews took place at the beginning and end of the research. At the end of the research process, three focus groups helped to validate the data gathered.

The sample of women who agreed to take part had not received reflexology before. This research seeks to establish whether or not reflexology is helpful in increasing feelings of well-being and alleviating stress.

By the end of the research, it was clear that many of the women had experienced a number of positive effects from the reflexology treatments. Approximately 80 percent of the sample experienced a reaction after the first one to five sessions. This was experienced as an emotional or physical effect. For example, one woman cried for three days, and several women had an increase in digestive problems such as flatulence.

In complementary therapies, such initial reactions are generally accepted and viewed as a positive sign in that emotions are not repressed but expressed, and physiologically, the body releases toxic congestion. Many women reported feeling very relaxed and energized immediately after their reflexology session.

There were a number of physical improvements including irritable bowel syndrome symptoms, the alleviation of back problems, premenstrual symptoms, and the improvement of headaches, appetite, sleep, and sinusitis. In one case, a woman's blood pressure was normalized, and for another her libido significantly increased. Underpinning these improvements were substantial increases in energy levels for many of the women. These physical improvements were reflected in a range of comments made by participants.

All the women showed significant improvements in their emotional state. One woman who reported at the beginning of the research process that she felt "despairing of life in general," stated at the end, "I feel more substantial . . . I feel I am more effective in the world. I feel like I'm in a hurricane world but it does not affect me. I'm like a tree that bends in the wind."

A common theme was the feeling that although their lives had not changed, the women were able to cope much better with potentially problematic situations.

One woman in her seventies described how she woke up in the morning feeling sixteen years old and tried to leap out of bed, only to be painfully reminded of her physical disability from osteoarthritis.

Others stated: "I found it very balancing, on the days I was down it uplifted me; on the days I was too up it brought me down." "Reflexology has done more for me than anything else anyone has done." "If I was very low it would have helped me more than doctors." "I feel like a tree that's grown long roots, I'm feeling much stronger and beginning to trust my own feelings and who I am. I feel more in control."

Many of the women reported an increase in self-esteem and confidence. Several also spoke of the way they were able to be more assertive with authority figures.

All participants agreed that reflexology made them feel relaxed and helped to alleviate anxiety states. They reported finding it easier to recognize their stress threshold and were actively attempting to alleviate the stress symptoms by employing relaxation techniques.

The women valued the sessions enormously, not only because it was a time for individual attention, but because of the importance of being listened to and heard by the reflexologist.

The experience of reflexology appeared to change the women's perceptions about themselves, e.g., being more accepting of their situations, feeling more empowered, valuing themselves, and becoming more assertive. The change in mood and perceptions of themselves, bearing in mind the evidence available, may therefore be responsible for improvements and alleviation of physical complaints reported during the study.

It would appear that reflexology was helpful in reducing and alleviating stress levels and symptoms and increasing feelings of well-being in the samples of women studied.

If reflexology can be used in conjunction with conventional allopathic approaches, there may be a reduction in drug dependency. This then represents a human cost reduction in relation to the attainment of positive and empowering health for the individual. It also represents an economic cost in relation to the savings accumulated on reduced purchasing of pharmaceutical drugs. A recent reflexology project in Denmark has demonstrated a significant annual savings for the Post Offices in Odense of approximately £110,000 (S. Madsen and J. Anderson, 1993, in *Association of Reflexologists Reflexology Research Reports*, 1996.)

Peta Trousdell

Association of Reflexologists, yoga teacher

Making Connections

(This is a summary of an evaluation of a complementary health-care project at Worthing Mind Day Centre (UK) by Peta Trousdell and Andrea Uphoff-Chmielnik. The following extract forms only part of an extensive study into the benefits of counseling and reflexology. A full copy of the above research report can be obtained from The Mind Day Centre in Worthing, England.)

This research was carried out between May 1996 and August 1997. Qualitative data collection methods were employed by a reflexologist and counselor in order to elicit user views and to monitor the safety and efficacy of both types of treatments. The reflexologist and the counselor worked with a total of seventy-four people over this period. Listed below are the key findings of the research from both the reflexology and counseling samples.

Physical improvements underpinned feelings of enhanced well being for many participants. For example, it was often remarked that the release of tension through being able to talk led to greater physical relaxation. This was found beneficial in the alleviation of headaches and an improved sleep cycle. A further reduction of other physical disturbances were noted by the counselor and reflexologist. For example, the counselor noted a decrease in hyperventilation and stuttering, the reflexologist found that a range of problems such as back problems, headaches, and digestive imbalances were often alleviated. Insights achieved through counseling and reflexology were occasionally responsible for life changes that had positive physical effects.

Many participants reported that an improved emotional status was established. The fear, worry, and despair reported at the beginning of counseling and reflexology were felt to have changed into more positive and fulfilling emotions. The reflexologist noted that participants appeared to "open up" emotionally during their reflexology sessions. A progressive ability to distinguish and differentiate emotions was observed by the counselor.

Underpinning the improvements reported in the reflexology sample were a significant increase in energy levels for most of the participants. Some participants remarked on their decreasing fear of exploration of emotions and choices. Some participants acknowledged the importance of touch, especially being touched in a safe and nonintrusive/nonabusive way during the reflexology sessions.

With the exception of two participants in the reflexology sample, there was a reported increase in relaxation levels and a decrease in anxiety levels. Most of the participants reported an increase in concentration levels, feeling more focused, and an increased ability to read a book, listen to music, or use a computer.

For many, motivation levels increased substantially. This was reported as being expressed in activities such as yoga, swimming, and other forms of exercise.

A substantial increase in self-esteem and confidence levels was reported by many of the participants. A common effect was that well-being levels increased for many. Participants reported finding an inner peace and were managing to "stay in the moment" rather than worry about the past or the future.

Some of the participants noted an increase in assertiveness in themselves and in others. This manifested itself in an ability to deal with difficult situations. A felt effect was that of being stronger and more in control.

Communication appeared to improve for some. Participants spoke of an ability to articulate ideas and express emotions and feelings more readily than was previously possible.

The counseling and reflexology processes became transparent for several participants, and they were able to ascertain how counseling and reflexology had worked for them. During counseling, participants reported being able, in some cases, to identify their own patterns of behavior and defense mechanisms. A reduction of obsessive behaviors was also remarked upon by a few. Many participants reported to the reflexologist the perceived energy flowing through the body, which mirrors acupuncture meridian theory.

The reflexologist noted that participants developed an increased awareness of tension in the body and an increased ability to change that state, e.g., they consciously altered their breathing, their posture, or listened to relaxing music as they became more aware of their emotional and physical tension. The counselor noted that self-awareness and awareness of others appeared to be an outcome of counseling for many of the participants. Many felt life had more opportunities than they had previously realized. Clarity was a feature reported many times. This was often accompanied by the ability to drop a social facade.

Many of the participant's felt that they were generally more balanced, and it appeared that for differing amounts of time homeostasis was achieved. Several participants reported being more able to feel, assess, and fulfill their own needs. They felt they were valuing themselves more, for example, by creating time for things they enjoyed and by cooking nutritious and balanced meals for themselves.

Often acknowledged was an ability to establish more satisfactory relationships and manifest more socially oriented behaviors. Some reported feeling strong enough to support others less fortunate. Others felt more robust in their interaction with authority figures. More boundaries between self and others were recognized and established.

Sensitivity issues were raised by a number of participants. Some felt that the professionals had very little time for them. Others felt not heard or, in some situations, overridden. In particular, a lack of information and choice within the services was criticized. Some participants were able to reduce or stop their medication mostly through cooperation with medical practitioners. Occasionally, participants reported having stopped medication themselves. This effect was not encouraged by the counselor or reflexologist. There was a general consensus among the participants that an offer of more complementary therapies would be of overall benefit within the mental health service.

Empowerment was felt and expressed by a number of participants. They reported this in terms of a newly found realism in their attitude toward life and their mental well-being. This, they felt, gave them more autonomy and trust in themselves.

Some participants described the benefits of experiencing both reflexology and counseling together. It appears that there may be a strong case for offering dual treatment when the advantages of the symbiotic relationship between counseling and reflexology can be utilized.

Peta Trousdell and Andrea Uphoff-Chmielnik

Authors note: Many thanks to Simon Duncan at the Association of Reflexologists UK for his kind assistance in helping contact many of the contributors in this chapter. The association is a well-known and respected reflexology organization based in the UK.

8

Disease and the Mind

This chapter examines some simple concepts and ideas on the subjects of health and healing from a Buddhist perspective. It is hoped that they are thought-provoking and stimulate debate among those interested in the field of complementary therapies. There is no intention to challenge religious beliefs. These ideas and theories are simply what I have found to be helpful in understanding and improving my own healing practice. We can apply them to our own lives or we can share them with our reflexology patients, friends, family, or anyone we meet who might benefit from some good advice.

Healthy Mind, Healthy Body

Nowadays many people are coming to the conclusion that the body and the mind cannot be separated in terms of understanding the cause and cure of ill health. Conventional medicine has for a long time ignored this vital and important link, choosing to look at the health of the patient from a purely physical perspective. There is really no doubt that the body and mind have an intimate, dependent relationship, and that good physical health is closely related to good mental, emotional, and spiritual health.

As mentioned in chapter 1, our thoughts and feelings arise and ride on subtle internal energies. So as physical illness is directly related to the quality of our internal energies, the predominant negative state of mind that accompanies an illness can be regarded as a symptom of the negative internal energy that is creating the conditions for the illness to manifest. We cannot say that the negative state of mind is the cause of the illness, as many New Age thinkers believe. If this were true, then everyone with a particular negative state of mind would develop the same illness or at least some illness. Also everyone with a positive state of mind would never become ill, but this is obviously not the case. We could say that, along with poor quality internal energies, negative minds are a "condition" that encourages illness to arise. However, as will be explained later on, we need to look deeper within the nature of the mind to discover the actual cause of illness.

Because of the close dependent relationship of our internal energies and our mind, we can say that each directly affects the other. Positive states of mind encourage and create healthy internal energies and visa versa. As physical health is directly related to the quality of our internal energies, therefore it is also directly affected by our thoughts and emotions.

We can prove this by simple logical reasoning. Some people can remain perfectly happy and content while experiencing poor health and even in the face of death when the internal energies that create good health have become weak and impure. Also plants and trees can develop diseases and die, resulting from poor internal energies, and they have no mind or consciousness. This shows that life force energy has a direct influence on health, and that the accompanying mind, although not a cause of illness, can have an influence on health by prolonging or shortening an illness or by influencing its severity. Again, there is much evidence to support this; for example, we know that our immune system is directly affected by our state of mind, and that people with long-term illnesses stand a much better chance of improving if they have a positive outlook. This mental influence is greatly increased if we can use our mind to consciously improve our internal energies through positive thinking and meditation. What actually causes poor quality energy to arise and encourage illness will be examined later when we look at the laws of karma, the root cause of all our problems and good fortune.

The way in which the various internal energies or subtle winds, as they are called in Buddhism, affect and control physical and mental health is a very detailed area for study. There are Buddhist texts available that fully explain this fascinating subject (see appendix 3), however, we do not need a detailed knowledge of this to be a good healer.

Transform What You Cannot Cure

Buddha said that "illness has many good qualities." This is true if we can transform what we cannot cure into the path to inner happiness. Often illness dispels pride and helps us develop such qualities as patience and contentment. Serious illness really concentrates the mind. It can certainly make us think more deeply about what we value in life and help us to reassess our priorities, attitudes, and lifestyle. Of course, no one would recommend "learning from illness" as a path of choice, but there are so many examples of people whose lives have been positively transformed simply by learning to look at themselves and their lives in a new light.

This may seem like a strange philosophy for a therapist or healer to share with their clients when so many people prefer to view illness as something to fight against with all your energy. Unfortunately, there are many instances when projecting too much energy at a problem by being blindly or unrealistically positive will just make things worse. We have to strike a balance in our approach to health and illness. Be realistic but positive, deal with the day-to-day reality of being ill, but don't rule out miracles. The people who learn to wisely adapt and learn to live with long-term illness are living examples of a life well spent, however short. Rare qualities like contentment, self-acceptance, inner calm, and compassion toward other's suffering can be developed over time. Such qualities are sometimes hard to find in those who appear to be successful and healthy. Hard times can really bring out the best in us if we are willing to use them to train our mind and transform our outlook.

So we can see that illness is not necessarily a negative force; in fact, it can be just the opposite. Simply by changing our mind, we can transform illness or any adverse condition into a meaningful opportunity to develop our own inner qualities. We never know what life is going to throw at us, but we can be ready for it if we are willing to be flexible, positive, and willing to accept difficulties and use them to become more whole and healthy human beings.

Healthy or Happy?

This raises the question, "What is good health?" Is it a healthy body or a healthy mind? Many New Age thinkers would say that it is a balance between the two, but if we think deeply about this, we can see that good health is simply a state of mind. Some people have developed the capacity to be deeply happy and content in the most adverse situations. Dealing with great physical or environmental difficulties and becoming stronger, more whole, and complete human beings because of it. Such people often become spiritually and mentally healthy—perhaps more healthy, in the truest sense of the word, than Olympic athletes! Certainly, our inner achievements are ultimately of more value than our external triumphs. Although their value is not as immediately obvious, they are a real treasure, and if we build on them and strive to develop our inner qualities, we will find great peace and contentment in this life and far into the future.

Although material wealth and good health give us a sense of security, this will be short lived. Sooner or later these things will be taken from us, and certainly at the end of our life we will have to leave them behind. There is no reason why we should not enjoy these short-term pleasures, but if we expect them to afford some lasting comfort and protection, we will be disappointed. So we have to look elsewhere for some lasting happiness and security, and the best place to start is within. What we gain from within, what we learn about ourselves, what good qualities we develop as we go through life will always be with us. If we are happy within, our outlook will be positive whatever our circumstances. If we can share this point of view with patients, clients, friends, family, or anyone we meet, either directly or through good example, we are really giving them something of great value. To give this kind of wisdom is the wisest kindness.

A Simple Antidote

So often the simple antidote to future illness is to "stop and think" before illness makes you stop and think! Giving yourself regular time and space to look at your life and the way you are living it is really important. Regular meditation, prayer, walks in the country—whatever helps you to get in touch with yourself and develop a little wisdom and clarity—is priceless. It helps us to see where we are going and what might be coming to meet us in the future. It is not as difficult to see into the future as we think. It is simply a task of knowing that if we do not change our way of living and being, then the past will tend to repeat itself, and the future is generally a simple projection of the present. If our life is gray and dull now, it will probably be gray and dull, or worse, in the future, especially if we do not make an effort to paint a little "color" into things.

We cannot buy these inner qualities, yet they are of the highest value. No one can give them to us, and, fortunately, no one can take them away. We have to make an effort to develop them and keep them. This can be achieved most easily if we are walking a spiritual path or a path to personal growth that is authentic, complete, tried, and tested. If we try to succeed alone or if we choose a path that is not genuine, we may progress intermittently but eventually we may find we slip back into our old patterns of negativity and self-doubt. Having someone special to guide us and support our progress and others to compare notes and share the journey with is a great help and a guarantee of success.

Being happy is an art that many of us have forgotten. Many people are discontent and possess great inner poverty, even the rich and famous. Yet it is not difficult to find happiness within when someone points us in the right direction. Developing inner happiness and contentment is a great treasure that we can all have in abundance simply by understanding and changing our inner nature. In fact, all we really need is a happy mind. Understanding the true causes of happiness and suffering is right at the heart of Buddhist philosophy. If you are interested in knowing more about this, it is best to read appropriate books or consult a fully qualified teacher (see appendices 2 and 3).

Many of the healing techniques that Buddha taught and practiced are still used to this day, including the well-known practices of the Medicine Buddha, the embodiment of all the Buddha's healing qualities. We can receive the empowerment of Medicine Buddha from a qualified Buddhist teacher, which can help us to create a special connection with this healing Buddha. We can then receive teachings on a simple meditation practice in order to use the blessings of the Healing Buddha to heal ourselves and others. Again, consult appendix 2 if you wish to know more about this from a qualified teacher.

Creating Your Own Reality

We all live in a slightly different universe! Obviously, animals experience a different world than humans, but every human also experiences the outside world in a different way. We have different personal perceptions of the same phenomena caused by having different minds. For example, when we are young, we may not like curry, but as we grow older, we may change our mind and stop perceiving curry as a source of displeasure. We may actually begin to see curry as a great source of pleasure. In this instance, we can see that curry has not changed; it was never inherently good or bad. We can also apply this to any phenomena—that nothing is inherently good or bad. We project these qualities onto objects, people, places, etc., and then believe them to be real, as if these objects actually possess good or bad qualities within their make-up. Another good example is when we meet someone for the first time. We immediately form an opinion of them. However, that first opinion is often proved to be wrong, and we may easily grow to dislike or like that person given time.

So what relevance does this have to reflexology and other healing techniques? Well, simply this:

Peaceful mind = peaceful world

Complementary therapies should help us change our mind, not the world around us; by changing our mind, all things change. Our perception of ourselves, our environment, and others changes completely when we change our mind or when our mind is changed. This tried-and-tested ancient wisdom for solving all our problems can be summed up in one phrase:

All we need is a happy mind!

We will never find lasting happiness by trying to manufacture a perfect world for ourselves. We can try to find the best job, the right partner, the nicest house, or the fastest car, and for a short time we may find some happiness in these things, but if we are honest, we know in our hearts that this happiness will come to an end. It is not real happiness and often serves to create more problems than it solves. In fact, the amount of pain and unhappiness we experience when we are separated from these things will at the very least be proportionate to the amount of attachment we have to them. There is a strong relationship between need and pain. The more we need someone or something to make us happy, the more pain we will experience when we are eventually parted from them.

We also spend much time and effort manipulating our world to get what we want, when we want it, when all the happiness and peace of mind we could wish for is literally under our noses! As mentioned before, if we have a deeply happy mind, we can experience all manner of difficult circumstances and unpleasant situations and not feel any less happy. We also know that if we are deeply unhappy, no amount of money, possessions, or relationships can help us. So again, this shows us that happiness depends upon the mind, not on external factors. Understanding this simple wisdom and taking it to heart should give us great hope, because this realization is the root of great happiness and the essence of a true spiritual path. The door of the mind is the gateway to heaven.

Learning to open our hearts and minds and develop some simple wisdom and contentment is time well spent, and the rewards for accumulating these inner treasures are fathomless. This is not some difficult or mystical task; it is very simple and natural to all of us, and we can use complementary therapies to help us begin and complete this journey toward self-understanding and lasting peace of mind.

To walk a path of spiritual or personal growth does not mean we have to shave our heads and run to the hills! This would be an extreme and another way of trying to manipulate our world to avoid what we dislike. The real spiritual practitioner realizes that they have exactly the right conditions at present to start developing higher qualities within themselves. Whether we are rich or poor does not matter. What matters is that we make an effort to change from within. Simply making a daily determination to be a little more tolerant, patient, kind, and helpful is a great step forward. Then if we can carry forward these determinations into our daily activities and remind ourselves of our good intentions, especially when we are challenged by our own impatience or selfishness, we will begin to make real progress.

Again, we may wonder what relevance all this has to reflexology. Well, if we want to be good healers or therapists, we need to understand what good health is. Then we will know how to help people achieve it. Is good health a physical or a mental, emotional, or spiritual quality. The outer practice of reflexology to be truly effective should be combined with the healer's inner qualities and knowledge of the human condition. Just being in the presence of a healer with a little wisdom and compassion is really of more benefit in the long term than a thousand hands-on treatments from someone who is in it for the money, recognition, or some other wrong motivation.

The Key to Success

Intention and motivation is the key to success. If our motives are good—even if we make mistakes—the results will be beneficial right from our very first treatment. It is also useful to remember that there is a right and a wrong time for giving advice. When people are not ready to change their minds and move toward good health, then bombarding them with well-intentioned advice can be a real turn-off—we all know this! Wisdom dictates that a gentle approach, patience, and a good listening ear need to be employed until a patient naturally seeks knowledge for a new perspective on an old problem. A wise farmer will not throw good seed on poor ground; when the ground is fertile, that is the right time to plant.

We have to also be careful that a sense of wisdom does not breed arrogance or some subtle sense of superiority. Some Eastern philosophies teach that the best healers are those that always regard the welfare of others, especially their patients, as most important. This sense of humility that many of the great spiritual teachers like Jesus and Buddha displayed is a very rare and great quality. It really allows us to get close to others and helps them to feel comfortable with us. A sense of superiority is a real barrier to the development of any healing relationship.

Conditions that Encourage and Prevent Illness

Regular reflexology can greatly enhance our health and protect us from future illness by preventing the potential causes of illness arising from deep within the mind. Illness can only arise from within the mind if the right conditions are present; for example, a seed cannot grow into a tree without water, earth, light, air, etc. Likewise, a potential illness can be prevented from arising by eliminating stress, poor diet, depressing environments, and, most importantly, negative states of mind and poor quality internal energies. Using reflexology can be a protection against a negative mind and impure internal energy, the major conditions that cause illness to arise. So reflexology can work in two ways: to heal existing problems and prevent future ones arising.

Karma—Actions and Their Effects

Basically we can say that any disease, disorder, or unhappiness is the result of some disharmony in the body, mind, or environment. However, it is not an easy task to establish the original cause of a particular problem. From Buddhism we know that the root causes of all our major and minor problems are our own previous negative actions of body, speech, and mind returning to us as illness, poverty, ignorance, or any other type of unpleasant experience. The word "karma" directly translates as "action" or what we intentionally create mentally, verbally, and/or physically. The laws of karma teach that whatever we create or give out comes back to us sooner or later, just like a boomerang. These negative actions may have been performed many lifetimes ago, and it is only now that we might be experiencing the effects or repercussions. We may think that we would never have committed serious negative actions like harming others, but in each of our previous lives we were almost completely different from the kind of person we are now. If we met ourselves from a previous life, we would not recognize ourselves at all. It would be like meeting a complete stranger.

Buddhism suggests that with each lifetime we are almost born anew. On the surface we have completely different bodies and personalities, yet deep within our very subtle mind, soul, or higher self we carry the memories, tendencies, and imprints of all our previous lives. When the conditions are right, our previous actions of body, speech, and mind will return to us as positive or negative experiences, depending on whether they were well-intentioned and beneficial or otherwise. So from a Buddhist perspective, to fully heal and prevent future illness, we must remove the root causes or the seeds of our past negative actions from deep within the mind, before they ripen as unpleasant experiences.

We could just as easily say that any person is simply the results of his or her previous actions ripening as pleasant or unpleasant characteristics and experiences. However, because one person is experiencing happiness and good fortune does not necessarily mean he or she is superior than others, or that they have been kinder or more giving in previous lives. We all have an infinite amount of accumulated karma, because we have had countless previous lives. We have all been good and bad people in previous lives, so we don't know what karma will ripen next; it might be pleasant it might not.

Unfortunately, karma ripens haphazardly. There is no grand plan or great scheme. Life is simply a "karmic lottery." If the conditions are right, any sort of karma could ripen, anything could happen to us. We know this is a fact of life. Bad things can happen to good people and vice versa. A murderer can be reborn as a king in his next life if he has the karma from a previous life for that to happen. He may experience many fortunate rebirths in wealthy and loving families until eventually the karma of murder catches up with him.

Fortunately, we can protect ourselves from our own negative karma by completely purifying it before it ripens and while we have the wisdom and opportunity to do so. We cannot escape the law of karma simply by not believing it. It is a fact of life—a universal law.

Liberation through Acceptance

Sometimes no matter how hard we try and no matter what therapies or remedies we use, we cannot escape or remove the effects of heavy negative karma that might be ripening in the form of a serious, possibly life-threatening, illness. This is a fact of life that can be difficult to accept. Of course, we can use reflexology and other therapies to help us deal with such challenging situations, but we also have to be realistic and mature. Sometimes we simply have to accept what is happening to us and stop fighting. Developing a peaceful and happy mind is possible even in the face of great hardship. Learning to accept the things we cannot change and developing compassion for others who may be feeling for us shows great wisdom and maturity. Also, accepting difficulties with a peaceful and patient mind actually causes negative karma to be purified and exhausted much more quickly than if we develop anger, frustration, or sadness. Of course, we may go through these emotions initially on the path to acceptance, but if we "stay there" too long, we are only making a difficult situation worse for ourselves and for those we love.

So from Buddhism we know that any illness, before manifesting on the physical or conscious level, initially arises from the very subtle or deepest levels of mind, which are presently subconscious to most people. Ultimately, we can only remove the true causes of illness by knowing, experiencing, and purifying our very subtle mind of all the potential seeds of illness planted or created by our own past negative actions in previous lives. This is our karma.

However, even when these seeds have ripened or been removed, the mental imprints of these past actions still remain in the mind, like footprints in the sand, and these create the mental tendencies to walk the same path again or commit similar negative actions in the future. These imprints must also be removed if we want to fully prevent illness or other negative experiences coming our way in this and future lives. We can do this by completely purifying our very subtle mind and developing a special type of wisdom, understanding the true nature of reality or, in other words, gaining enlightenment. Again, this is not some far-off, unattainable spiritual goal. The potential for us to achieve this is in our very nature. We just need someone to point us the right direction.

One tried-and-tested way toward enlightenment is through practicing the simple and clear meditation techniques that Buddha taught. We do not have to become Buddhist to learn these. They are open and available to anyone, and they are ideally suited to our needs whatever our circumstances and commitments. In fact, we do not need to change our lifestyle at all— only our mind.

Selfishness—The Source of All Suffering

As explained before, the main cause of illness is negative karma ripening when the correct conditions are in place. But what causes us to create negative karma?

The simple answer to this is that "our selfish mind causes us to create negative karma." Likewise, a selfless mind causes us to create positive karma that will come back to us as a pleasant experience in the future, and then we will also find it easier to repeat this tendency to be kind, thoughtful, and selfless again and again, bringing greater and greater good fortune and happiness.

Thinking of the welfare of others is a great source of future happiness, and thinking of our own welfare is a source of future suffering. Even in the short term, transferring our attention toward others and working for their benefit can take our mind off our own problems and cause us to be less introverted and self-obsessed. The more we worry about a problem, the bigger it gets, but the more we concern ourselves with helping others, the less energy and time we give to our own worries and the weaker and less demanding they become.

We can use this line of reasoning in many practical ways. For example, if we have to give a public talk on a particular subject, we may be very worried or frightened, especially if we have little experience. But if we change our mind, and instead of giving our attention to our own worry think, "How can I help these people?" "What can I give them?" Then by strongly concentrating on these thoughts, our own worries will naturally diminish. This line of reasoning is very powerful and can be applied to many situations that cause us unhappiness or worry.

One of our greatest sources of happiness and unhappiness is relationships, and again, simply by consistently concentrating on the welfare of the other person in a relationship, this will definitely help us to become more content and less demanding or controlling. All the great spiritual teachers have taught and encouraged this, they know that the source of all happiness is caring for others, all others, equally.

Putting others first does not mean we have to be hard on ourselves. On the contrary, if we understand and accept the laws of karma, we can gain great personal satisfaction from knowing that selfless actions not only benefit others but will also cause us to experience good fortune in the future. Also, the main factor in creating karma is our true intention or motivation. Many people might appear to be altruistic on the outside, always doing good turns for others, but if their motivation is selfish, perhaps because they want others to like them, then this will not create a good karmic return in the future. Conversely, leading a very normal life with pure motivation will lead to greater future happiness.

So we can say that illness arises from negative karma that was created by selfish actions in a previous life, but what causes us to perform selfish actions? What causes us to think and act in a selfish way? If we can understand the answers to these questions, then we are truly on the way to solving all our problems and finding a lasting cure to any present or potential future illness.

The Universal Cure

We act instinctively and naturally to benefit ourselves, because we think we are more important than others. Our sense of self is very dear to us, and we cherish it deeply and in many subtle ways. We do not realize how deeply we cherish ourselves until we are faced with situations that frighten or challenge our sense of self. So we have a strong sense of self, a strong sense that we truly exist, and that this self is the most important thing in the universe. The fact that we grasp at this sense of self, ego, or I, and believe it to truly exist, is the source of all our present and future problems. If we could realize our true nature and abandon the inner ignorance or lack of inner clarity/wisdom that gives rise to the sense of a very important self, we could solve all our problems and experience complete and lasting happiness and freedom from suffering forever. Again, this may sound unrealistic, unattainable, or even bizarre, but this message usually strikes a chord, even in the most cynical heart.

We can compare the mind to a glass of sparkling water; the constant stream of bubbles floating to the surface are like our thoughts and feelings. It appears that we "are" these thoughts and emotions that arise from within, as if they make up our identity and character, or as if they are the "real me." Our true nature is more like the water itself than the bubbles that arise in it. Our essence or source in reality is closer to the space between our thoughts and feelings.

Ultimately, this inner realization can become the universal cure for all illness and suffering.

So now having established a universal cure for all ills, how do we take it? How can we free ourselves and others from the effects of illness and the potential for future illness and all forms of suffering? The old biblical saying of "Physician, heal thyself" is very relevant here. We cannot truly help others until we have healed ourselves, and a true healing is one that is complete and lasting and comes from within. Again, we can only accomplish this by realizing our true nature and becoming all that we can be. Then we will have the wisdom and power to help others achieve the same state of complete happiness and permanent freedom from any kind of problem or unhappiness. To reach this special destination, we have to find a path that leads there clearly and directly.

Buddha taught such a path thousands of years ago. Many people realized his teachings then and found great happiness and inner peace as a result. Because we have an unbroken and pure lineage of these teachings and instructions, many people from all backgrounds and religions today are also finding this timeless wisdom invaluable and completely relevant to the problems they face. Ultimately, Buddhism is really "Truism." It simply tells us the way things are, the way things will be, and the way we can improve them. If you ever wanted to know who you are, why you're here, and where you're going, simply pick up a good book on Buddhism. It will be a map of reality! (See appendix 3 for a list of books on Buddhism.)

Having said that, Buddhism does not have a monopoly on the truth. Many of Buddha's teachings are reflected in all of the great world religions and spiritual paths to truth and happiness. We cannot say that one is superior or better than another. They all have good qualities and, perhaps, we can say that they are all leading in a similar direction and come from the same "nameless" source. As individuals we have to find one that we feel comfortable with and one that we feel shines clarity and truth.

Working toward and achieving our true nature is not a painful or monumental task; we all have the potential and right conditions to achieve spiritual enlightenment in one lifetime. It is said that it is easier to gain enlightenment in one lifetime than it is to achieve a human rebirth—so really we have already done most of the work. Also, if we miss this precious opportunity, it may not come around again for a very long time.

The Most Effective Healer

Can the power of our compassion affect our reflexology treatment? The simple answer to this is "yes!" But we may not be able to see this clearly. Again, the mind is quite a subtle object, and the effects of the thoughts and intentions that accompany our actions are not easily revealed unless we are familiar with our inner world. However, we can prove this in another way. If someone were to practice reflexology and they were in a very negative frame of mind, perhaps impatient or distracted and not that bothered about the welfare of the person they were treating, then this would obviously have a profound effect on the treatment. The client would sense this and not be at ease and leave with little faith in the treatment. We can see that many "doors" are already closing, and the chance of a successful treatment is reduced. Conversely, if the therapist has his or her client's best interests at heart and has a mind of great compassion, then this will naturally lead to a successful treatment, and also give the client confidence in the therapist and, therefore, the treatment.

We also have to look again at karma to gain some clarity on this issue. Obviously, the karma of the client and therapist is the key factor in the possibility of a successful treatment. There are two conditions that they can establish that will help the karma of a successful treatment to ripen. From the therapist's side, the mind of pure compassion is vital; from the patient's side, the minds of patience, faith in the therapist, therapy, or the healing "energy" and the wish to be well are also vital. Even if we only have a little of these qualities present, then that will give reflexology enough room to work well.

Also, if the patient can try to develop more compassion for others, this will also aid his or her own healing process. We may wonder why this is so. Well, the opposite of compassion is a selfish mind, and selfish minds are one of the conditions that can encourage the karma of illness to ripen. Conversely, a wish to use your life well and help others whenever possible will help the karma of good health to ripen. It is important to stress that this is not a guarantee of good health, many compassionate people suffer from illness; it is simply another "condition" that can influence health.

Whatever conditions we create, good and bad, karma can only ripen if we have created the causes by planting the seeds of this karma by our actions of body, speech, and mind in previous lives. This is why some very negative people never get ill and have long lives and why some very positive people get ill and sometimes die young. It is all about causes and conditions. If we have not created the causes to be ill, or we have removed them through inner purification, whatever conditions we create, we will not become ill.

There is one more advantage in trying to develop our compassion: If selfish actions lead to future suffering, then compassion must lead to great health and happiness in the future.

9

Simple Meditations

There are many different types of meditation. Most of them aim to relax the body and promote peaceful and positive states of mind. The benefits of regular meditation are now well-known. We gain improved health and well-being in many ways, levels of stress are greatly reduced, and positive, peaceful, and confident states of mind are easily generated. As healers or therapists, when we have some experience of the benefits of meditation, we can share this with others by teaching clients, friends, or family how to relax the body and mind and generate a positive outlook.

The beauty of teaching patients a simple relaxation technique is that if they can do this a little everyday in between reflexology treatments, this will greatly assist their mental, emotional, and physical healing. There are many scientific studies to validate the healing power of meditation alone. With regular meditation, among other benefits, many people report increased mental clarity, more energy, reduced levels of stress, and a feeling of inner peace. So it can be as good for the therapist as for the patient.

Meditation is a very simple, natural, and powerful way of realizing our abilities to become more whole, healthy, and happy human beings from within. Meditation is not difficult, and it does not take years, months, or even weeks to master. We can receive great benefit, even from our very first meditation session. To gain the most from meditation, we really need to find a local meditation group that is led by an experienced teacher from an authentic tradition.

However, this chapter is designed to give you an introduction to meditation, and if you follow the instructions carefully, you can gain great benefit from practicing for just ten to fifteen minutes per day.

Meditation for Relaxation

This can be done either sitting up or lying down. Relaxing music may help, and you will need fifteen or twenty minutes of free time.

Begin by making a conscious intention to completely relax your body and mind and receive whatever healing you need during the time you have available for your greatest good. Take some deep breaths and settle into a comfortable position. Try to let go of anything that might be on your mind. This is your time to relax properly, and it's important that nothing distracts you.

Bring your attention to your toes and try to "find" any tension and release it. At first it may be helpful to tense and then release them. You need to gradually familiarize yourself with the experience of consciously relaxing, and then the process will become easier.

Move your attention slowly into the rest of your feet, consciously relaxing each part. If it helps, you can think "release and relax" as you slowly bring your attention to the ankles, shins, calves, knees, etc. Continue to move your attention up through the body, consciously relaxing each part. If your attention wanders, simply return to where you were.

When you have reached the top of your head, spend a few minutes being aware of how it feels to be completely relaxed. The more you remember this experience, the easier it will become to repeat and carry forward into your daily activities. This technique can take some time to master, so don't be disappointed if you still feel some tension after the first few sessions. This will pass in time and the technique will become natural.

At this point you can stop, dedicate your positive energy, and get up slowly, or you can continue with a simple visualization, such as the one that follows.

A Healing Visualization

Visualize a spiraling stream of golden or white light entering through the crown of your head, filling every part of your body. Try to move the light slowly down, so you get a sensation that each part of your body and every cell is filled with "light" energy. You can then imagine that your whole body and mind melts into this light, which slowly expands to fill the room, the house, town and country, the whole planet, and finally, the whole of space. Then spend some time enjoying this experience of pure light filling the whole of space.

If you wish, this is a good point to think of others who may need healing, of local or world conflicts, disasters, or simply "every living being." Visualize these people or situations surrounded by the light, and imagine that all their problems are easily transformed and healed. Then just continue to visualize them as healthy, happy, and content for a few minutes. You can think, "How wonderful, these people are now actually free from their pain and problems." Try to really believe that this has happened. Then concentrate for as long as possible on the feeling of joy that arises from this thought.

Don't worry if at first this feels false or manufactured. With sincere, regular practice, your motivation will become more natural and powerful. Also, don't try too hard or make your visualizations too complicated. An honest intention and a strong belief that your positive thoughts have really helped is the most important aspect.

The power of the mind is limitless. By strongly imagining that through your actions people are released from their problems, this creates the causes for it to actually happen in the future.

When you have finished, visualize the light coming slowly back into the space of your body, and seal it in with a mental intention such as:

> *Balanced, centered, grounded, blessed, and
> protected.*

Or think of something similar or even simpler. Then get up slowly when you are ready and dedicate the positive energy you have created. Sometimes when you are setting intentions like the one above, or dedicating the positive energy created through a healing action, it may helpful to say or think the intention three times. This sets the intention firmly in your mind and helps you to see if the intention sounds or feel right. It may be too complicated or not clear enough. You can change an intention simply by saying or thinking a new one that applies to the same person or situation. This will automatically override the previous one—if it is for the "greatest good."

The power of your intentions and dedications are dependent upon the sincerity and stability of your true heartfelt wishes, so you need to keep an eye on them and check them regularly.

Meditation for Developing Compassion

You prepare for this meditation by setting aside a regular, daily quiet time, about fifteen to twenty minutes or more. Early morning is often the best, when you are fresh. This can really help you start the day in a positive way.

The room you use should be peaceful and clean. If you have a particular religious affiliation, you can set up a small shrine or altar with holy pictures, scriptures, or offerings. This serves as a spiritual focal point and helps to build and hold a good quality of energy in the room and house, which is symbolic of your own body and mind. If you also intentionally honor, clean, and look after this space regularly and treat it with respect, you are definitely creating the causes for your meditations to gradually become clearer and deeper, with long-lasting benefits.

By inviting the universal blessings or "greatest good" into your house and life, and by creating a small shrine, you may also notice many positive benefits in other areas of your life. Other people may even comment that your house always seems peaceful and welcoming.

You can meditate sitting in a chair with your back straight, but not tense, your feet flat on the floor and hands resting in your lap. Or you can sit on a floor cushion in a traditional meditation posture.

For this meditation, relax the body and focus the mind by slowly mentally scanning the body for tension and releasing it. Begin at the top of your head and slowly work down through the various parts of the body until you reach the toes.

Bring your attention to your breathing and particularly to the sensation at the tip of the nostrils, as you feel the cool air coming in and the warm air as you breath out. Focus on this sensation completely. Your breathing is the "object" of meditation. This focuses the mind and improves your clarity and concentration. In fact, this simple breathing meditation, if practiced for ten to fifteen minutes daily, can help improve your quality of life by giving you a clear and peaceful mind. If you "lose" your object of meditation and begin thinking about other things, simply bring your attention back to the sensations of breathing.

If you have no experience with meditation, it can be helpful to practice just the breathing meditation for several days or even weeks before trying anything else.

There are two parts to the next stage of meditation: contemplation and placement. Contemplation is the mental process of considering the benefits of abandoning negative thoughts and actions and of adopting positive ones. When, as a result of this reasoning, a strong wish arises in the mind to change your behavior for the better, then this is your object of placement, and you should hold it or experience it for as long as possible.

To develop compassion, you can first contemplate how the opposite of compassion—anger and hatred—causes so many problems in the world. In fact, as mentioned earlier in the book, the selfish mind of anger is responsible for all conflicts and wars. If no one ever experienced anger, we would live in a very peaceful world.

Contemplate how angry or selfish thoughts and feelings have caused many problems and great unhappiness in the past, and consider how wonderful it would be to be free from these heavy, negative minds. When you naturally feel a strong wish to release these feelings and develop the opposing positive qualities, try to stay with and encourage these positive intentions.

Then contemplate the problems that others experience in their lives. You can think about people you know who are very unhappy, or you can think about situations you have heard about or read in the news, where people or animals are suffering. When a feeling of compassion arises in the mind toward these beings, hold onto it for as long as possible, and try to mix your mind with it completely, almost as if you have become completely compassionate and that is your true nature. We can think, "How wonderful it would be if all living beings were completely free from suffering."

Then make a firm determination or commitment to yourself to act to help others whenever and in whatever way you can. This determination is the final goal of your meditation. You should try to make it as deep and heartfelt as possible. Try to remember that determination throughout the rest of the day.

For a Successful Meditation

The key to successful meditation is to consistently make a strong inner determination to let go of negative and damaging ways of living and being, and develop more positive, harmonious, and constructive ones.

If your mind wanders during meditation, simply return to the contemplation until that strong wish to develop your good qualities arises again; then stay with that determination. You are actually training or encouraging yourself to eventually think and feel this way naturally. When you "hold" an object of meditation, you should not strain the mind; it should feel natural, as if your mind has completely mixed or become one with the object of meditation, i.e., your wish to be more tolerant, patient, or compassionate. By regularly developing these deep wishes to change for the better, you will definitely become more positive, happy, content, and considerate.

This ancient tried-and-tested way of dealing with life's problems, if practiced correctly and regularly, is a guaranteed solution, and unlike other modern methods of finding happiness, addiction to it produces very healthy results!

The meditations will also be most effective if you apply them directly to your own life based on your own life experiences. There is no point meditating everyday on a vague wish to love others if in your heart you are not really interested in changing, or if these meditations are not directly relevant to your life. It is possible to use the technique of meditation in this way to actually suppress or avoid your most relevant personal problems, thereby actually deepening these problems, and this is, of course, not meditation.

You have to mentally make the meditations come alive, and then carry your good intentions forward into the rest of the day. You do this by remembering the positive feelings and determination that arose during your meditation, and try to use this motivation to guide all your actions of body and mind. Whenever you become aware that negative feelings or thoughts, like worry or impatience, are about to arise in the mind, you can prevent them from influencing you by recalling your earlier good intentions. In this way, your wisdom and happiness will gradually increase, and your daily problems will steadily decrease.

Toward True Wisdom

One of the special qualities of authentic meditation is that it increases wisdom. Wisdom is very different from intellectual ability. Many intelligent people are very unhappy. Since all living beings have the same basic wish to avoid problems and find happiness, wisdom is simply the ability to understand where lasting happiness comes from. As you meditate daily, you will come to see that happiness is simply a state of mind, and that since you have the opportunity to create positive states of mind through meditation, prayer, etc., these methods are the key to lasting happiness.

Although the essence and practice of meditation is fairly simple, it is a good idea to seek out a qualified and experienced teacher who can guide you along the path of meditation. If you try to learn on your own or from a book, you may encounter problems and waste time. Consequently, you can lose interest because you are not experiencing consistently good results. Learning and sharing your experiences with others, meditating in a group and having the opportunity to ask questions can greatly assist your enjoyment and progress. Also, having a teacher who is a living example of what you can achieve through meditation is a constant inspiration and encouragement to your own development.

If you do a little meditation every day, good results will accumulate. You will become more relaxed and more able to enjoy life fully. Gradually, you will become a true source of wisdom, compassion, and inner strength!

10

The Future of Reflexology

Possibly one of the best aspects of reflexology is that anyone can practice it successfully and effectively. If you have no intention to practice professionally, you can use books like this one to learn the techniques to give good, effective treatments to friends and family and anyone else interested in experiencing the benefits of this wonderful therapy for the body and mind. If there was just one person who could practice reflexology in every family or circle of friends everywhere, this would have a profound effect on world health and well-being.

This is what we need to aim for. This is the future of reflexology. We do not need lots of new and fancy techniques; the basics are tried and tested and, without a doubt, work wonders. Of course, new developments are good. Anything that serves to improve our ability to help others through reflexology should be taken seriously. But the real message that we need to acknowledge is that the best reflexologist is not the most technically proficient but simply the most compassionate and understanding person that he or she can be. This might be a controversial issue, but we cannot ignore the fact that this means the best reflexologists might not be professionally qualified. They might not be widely known or famous. In fact, they might just so love what they are able to do for family and friends, in a quiet way, that they themselves do not realize their own value.

The Meaning of Illness

Hard times are never meaningless if you know how to transform them to develop your inner qualities. From the point of view of dealing with illness, one of the most valuable qualities you can develop or help others develop is patience, which reduces your/their propensity for anger and frustration.

As mentioned earlier, Buddha said that "illness has many good qualities." There is no doubt that many people would strongly disagree with this. How can any form of suffering be beneficial? We all work constantly to avoid suffering and find happiness. However, if we check, the happiness we seek in the external world is transient and provides no lasting satisfaction; often the temporary happiness we find in relationships and possessions only leads to greater unhappiness when we are parted from them. But the happiness that comes from a peaceful and contented mind can never be stolen and will never leave us, even when we die.

Many people develop such happiness by learning to live with and transforming illness into the "inner path." There are many instances of this happening, and it does raise the question "What is the value of healing if it denies us the opportunity to develop such inner wisdom and happiness?" Obviously, we do not have to be ill to develop such qualities, but such circumstances can point us in the right direction. Then when we are familiar with that path and no longer need an illness to point us in the right direction, then that can be an appropriate time for healing. Again, there is no guarantee of this, but it often happens this way.

As a healer, the most important lesson to learn from all this is that although you want people to be healthy, your main aim should be to help people make the most of the opportunities they have to find some lasting happiness now and in the future. This will only come about through realizing their own divinity or spiritual nature—not necessarily through good health and success in the external world. These are simple but challenging truths.

One more interesting result of trying to develop your spiritual qualities is that you are able to enjoy your relationships and external possessions much more when you reduce your attachment and need for them. It is as if the less you need these things, the more fun we have! Having more space and clarity in your mind helps you to view the external world in a more playful and less serious way, while your regard for the really serious issues, like your wish for others to be happy, increases.

The final question these issues raise is "Are we as healers/therapists willing to acknowledge these truths and live our lives as a good example to the people we are trying to help?" Well, we do not have to be perfect, but there is no reason why we shouldn't try!

Dedication

To the greatest benefit for all living beings.

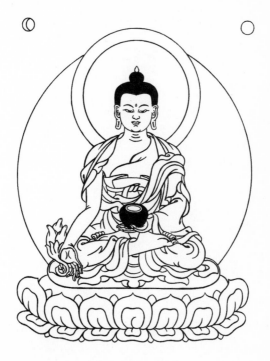

Medicine Buddha

Appendix 1:
The History of
Reflexology

The roots of reflexology are vague and generally not well-known. We know that many ancient civilizations practiced some form of foot therapy for health and relaxation, but the extent to which those practices relate to modern reflexology is unclear. In fact, modern reflexology was discovered and developed independently, without any apparent foundation or basis in the ancient forms of foot therapy.

This in itself is quite remarkable, and some people have speculated that the founders of modern reflexology might have subconsciously remembered practicing foot therapy in a previous life. This has simply been redeveloped and explained in a modern context. This idea is supported by the Buddhist belief in reincarnation and the tendency of the mind to be attracted to those things with which it is familiar. For example, those people who have worked in the healing arts and sciences in previous lives are more likely to have an apparently natural or innate interest and attraction to those same vocations in this and future lives. The mind is a subtle mystery, and not many people, least of all modern psychologists/psychiatrists, understand its nature.

Unfortunately, this principle of attraction or habit also applies to those people who are attracted to negative, harmful, or criminal actions. If we cause harm to others, we will experience harm from others in the future, but we will also create a tendency or habit in the mind to naturally wish harm to others in the future. It is a simple matter of cause and effect.

No one is inherently good or bad; the true nature of the mind goes beyond such boundaries. No one and nothing stays the same. Negative habits that have been developed over many lifetimes can be overcome in one lifetime. We all have infinite potential to become someone or something very special. The act of true healing should set us on this course.

It is interesting to note that all the ancient civilizations that practiced foot therapy accepted the laws of karma as the natural laws of the universe, and individuals lived their lives in accordance with these ancient teachings on how to live a happy and meaningful. When people from such countries come to the West, they are often genuinely shocked and saddened to see how Westerners live their lives, as they understand the kind of karma that these people are creating for their future lives.

The Eastern Connections

The most obvious and well-known of the ancient systems of foot therapy originated in China. It was developed as part of the therapies known today as acupuncture and acupressure. These therapies are known and respected for their effectiveness throughout the world. Briefly, they are based on the theory that within the human body there are many invisible pathways through which flow life force energies, or chi. When these pathways become blocked and the free flow of energy is restricted or unbalanced, then illness can result. Acupressure and acupuncture helps to release the blockages and stimulate the body's natural healing responses. All the major energy pathways run into the feet. As the feet are often sensitive and receptive to touch, they were thought to be especially important areas to treat as were the hands and the ears.

This is also borne out by two facts. First, we know from ancient Indian medicine that there are energy chakras on the soles of the feet. These chakras allow our energy system to soak up the life-giving and healing chi that the Earth naturally emits. Second, it makes sense that the body would develop or evolve sensitive reflexes on the soles of the feet since we naturally spend so much time walking or standing. The reflexes are naturally stimulated by these actions, and this has a corresponding positive effect on the body's energy system and the related physiological systems.

Although reflexology developed separately from any influence of acupuncture or acupressure, modern reflexologists take a great interest in these fields of knowledge and apply them to their practice. Although to become an accomplished reflexologist we do not need such knowledge, an awareness of meridian theory is useful and an understanding of life force energy can greatly improve our understanding of the healing process.

The oldest known documentation of reflexology is depicted on the wall of a tomb of an Egyptian physician called Ankmahor, located in Saqqara in Egypt. It dates back to around 2330–2500 B.C. and shows two men working on the feet of two other men. On the inscription the patient says, "Do not hurt me," and the therapist replies, "I shall act so you praise me."

There are several other similar pictographs from other dates showing that some form of reflexology was being practiced throughout Egypt. More often than not it is royalty or nobility being treated by the physicians or their assistants. This would indicate that the practice was probably quite widespread throughout the rest of society, especially as it didn't involve expensive medicines and was effective for relieving the effects of constant manual labor.

It is also thought that foot therapy was used in South America, possibly by the Incas, and that this was passed down to the Native American Indians. Many tribes believed that the connection to the Earth energies through the feet indicated that the feet were particularly special, and some form of foot therapy was used as part of their healing arts.

The Development of Zone Therapy

It is known that a type of pressure therapy was practiced in Europe as far back as the fourteenth century. Indeed, some books on the subject were written and published in the fifteenth and sixteenth centuries. In the 1890s, Sir Henry Head of London did extensive research into what he called "head zones." These were areas of skin connected by nerve tissues to diseased organs, which were very sensitive to touch.

Possibly the first person to apply massage to reflex zones was Dr. Alfons Cornelius. Around 1893 he suffered an infection, which led to him receiving a course of massage. He found that when he received massage on certain areas of the body, this had an increased healing action on his condition. When fully recovered, he pursued this line of research.

Despite many people having a knowledge or interest in some form of zone therapy or pressure points by the late eighteenth century, it was not until the beginning of this century that the theory of modern zone therapy was developed. Dr. William Fitzgerald pulled all these strands together in his research. Dr. Fitzgerald studied with interest the techniques a doctor from Vienna was researching, techniques for treating certain conditions with pressure points.

Dr. Fitzgerald began his own research into this area while working as the head physician at the Hartford Ear, Nose, and Throat Hospital in Connecticut. The first thing he discovered was that if constant pressure was applied to the fingers, it would create an anaesthetic effect in the hand, arm, shoulder, neck, and face on the same side of the body. With this numbing effect, he was even able to carry out minor surgery on these areas.

He further discovered that the body could be divided into ten vertical zones, running from head to toe, and corresponding to the ten fingers and ten toes. Pressure applied to certain fingers would have an effect on parts of the body contained within the corresponding zones.

The following section from the book *Zone Therapy* by Dr. Fitzgerald and Dr. Edwin Bowers, published in 1917, explains how Dr. Fitzgerald discovered and formulated his theories:

> *I accidentally discovered that pressure with a cotton tipped probe on the mucocutaneous margin of the nose gave an anaesthetic result as though a cocaine solution had been applied. I further found that there were many spots in the nose, mouth, throat, and on both surfaces of the tongue which, when pressed firmly, deadened definite areas of sensation. Also, that pressures exerted over any body eminence, on the hands, feet, or over the joints, produced the same characteristic results in pain relief. I found also that when pain was relieved, the condition that produced the pain was most generally relieved. This led to my "mapping out" these various areas and their associated connections, and also to noting the conditions influenced through them. This science I have named zone therapy.*

In 1915, Dr. Edwin Bowers, Dr. Fitzgerald's colleague, wrote an article for *Everybody's Magazine* titled "To Stop That Toothache Squeeze Your Toe!" This caused great interest, and many people became interested in zone therapy. The doctors often experienced skepticism from their medical peers and sometimes would prove their theories if the skeptic was brave enough. They would anesthetize an area of the skeptic's face by applying pressure to the relevant finger and then push a pin into the skin. This would quickly convert the skeptic into a believer.

A Case of Foot and Mouth

Another story showing the effectiveness of zone therapy was at a dinner party Dr. Fitzgerald was attending. He was asked what zone therapy could do for one of the guests who was a professional singer. The upper register of her voice had gone flat and this was causing her great concern. She had already consulted medical specialists who could not help her. Dr. Fitzgerald looked at her throat, and then, to the amusement of the other guests, he asked to look at the singer's hands and feet. After a short examination, he told her that her problem was caused by the formation of a callus on her right big toe. Again, this caused much amusement, but the doctor simply smiled and applied pressure to the callused area for a few minutes. The doctor then asked her to try the upper register of her voice. Not only was she able to easily reach the notes she had been missing, but she was able to reach two tones higher than she had ever done before.

Zone therapy was not developed further by Dr. Fitzgerald and Dr. Bowers, possibly because they thought there was not much more to be discovered but also much of what they had presented to the medical world was not regarded with much respect or interest. One doctor who did have a high regard for their work was Dr. Joseph Shelby Riley. Dr. Riley and his wife, Elizabeth, were taught zone therapy by Dr. Fitzgerald and applied it in their medical practice for many years. It was Dr. Riley who made the first detailed drawings and diagrams of the reflex points located on the feet. He also added to the ten vertical zones eight horizontal zones on the body, which made pressure treatment more accurate. He also wrote four books covering all aspects of zone therapy.

The Mother of Modern Reflexology

Dr. Riley had an assistant named Eunice Ingham (1879–1974), who is now widely regarded as the mother of modern reflexology. She believed that it was the feet alone that held the greatest potential for healing through zone therapy. Eunice spent many years researching and developing techniques, which transformed the fairly basic and unrefined methods of zone therapy into the technically detailed, powerful, and complete healing practice we know today as reflexology.

Although she was trained by Dr. Riley in zone therapy, she began to feel that as the feet were such sensitive areas of the body they might, through some form of applied pressure or massage, hold the key to a deeper, gentler, and swifter form of healing therapy. Her intuitions were proved to be correct, and when she began to gain excellent results through her work, this fired her enthusiasm and set her on the way to developing a systematic therapy that anyone could learn in order to help others. She was particularly enthusiastic about sharing her knowledge with nonmedical or lay practitioners in the hope that many people would learn her techniques and practice on friends and family. She was not bothered about recognition from the medical profession, as she had seen the way they had reacted to zone therapy. She knew that the methods she was developing were effective for relieving and healing all manner of conditions, and she simply wanted many people to benefit from this knowledge.

Through her research, she discovered that the whole body could be mapped out through the reflexes on the feet, as if the feet were a mirror of the whole body. As the excellent results of her work continued, word spread and people from miles around came to see her and receive treatments. Eunice's nephew Dwight Byers recalls that during 1935, she was developing and practicing her new therapy in a small village on Conesus Lake in New York. Dwight received many treatments for his asthma and hay fever, and his aunt talked to him during those treatments about her work and how her research was developing. Today Dwight runs the International Institute of Reflexology.

Spreading the Good News

When Eunice's methods became widely known, she began to travel throughout America, giving talks and lectures, and teaching her methods to many people. She also wrote two books, which are seminal texts for all those interested in practicing reflexology: *Stories The Feet Can Tell* (1938) and *Stories the Feet Have Told* (1963). If Eunice could be aware of the extent to which her work has benefited others and has been embraced by millions of people worldwide, she would be very pleased.

Reflexology has not replaced zone therapy. Indeed, many reflexologists use it as a useful aid to the healing process, and the client or patient can easily be taught to use this therapy between regular reflexology treatments. Many reflexologists also combine other therapies with their practice, like reiki, aromatherapy, and the Bach Flower Remedies. These are all excellent and complementary additions to the healing program, which all modern therapists should seriously consider using.

What's New in Reflexology

Many reflexologists also consider it important to have a knowledge of Chinese meridian theory, and some believe that the explanations this gives for how foot massage stimulates healing is more accurate than that provided by zone therapy. In fact, we could say that the knowledge we have gained from meridian theory has taken reflexology forward since the discoveries of Dr.

Fitzgerald and Eunice Ingham. Meridian theory is quite an in-depth subject and principally derived from what we know about acupuncture and Chinese medicine. There are many books available on these subjects, which the interested reflexologist could easily access.

For the moment, though, it is interesting to note that reflexology is really nothing new. Many ancient civilizations were far more medically advanced than our own. They understood the subtle energies of the body and the implications that mental and emotional well-being have on physical health. They then developed their healing techniques accordingly. We have lost much of this precious wisdom, and modern medicine, although very valuable, sometimes blindly pursues healing from a purely physical standpoint. Most of us need to see physical evidence of anything before we believe that the "unseen" might exist. We are afraid to trust our other senses, especially the subtle ones like intuition and inner wisdom. However, gradually, some people are beginning to open their eyes and consider the possibilities that there may be other ways to health and happiness, other than purely conventional medicine and materialism. So with reflexology, we are not discovering anything new—only finding our feet again.

There is no doubt that reflexology, like other complimentary therapies, will not stand still. New developments will come and should be embraced once tried and tested. A good therapist should always be open to new ideas while being cautious of so-called miracle cures. There is a vast amount of information about reflexology available, much of which is published on the Internet. For the new practitioner it is probably not worth getting bogged down in all this. A good reflexologist doesn't have to know the ins and outs of all the theories and developments, especially if they only intend to practice on friends and family. There is much to be said for just studying a few well-chosen books and practice, practice, practice. Apart from this, a good healer is naturally a good healer. If you have it in you, it will come out. Of course, the more effort you apply, the more easily your healing qualities will arise naturally from within.

Appendix 2: Meditation Groups

The demand for a lasting solution to the problems of stress and anxiety, created by the nature of today's materialistic society, has led to the creation of meditation groups in many towns and cities. These groups vary in content and in their spiritual origin, so it is important to find one that you feel comfortable with; one that is run by a fully qualified teacher, and one that teaches a recognized and correct "path" true to the origins of meditation.

Buddhist Meditation

Most meditation groups can trace their origins back to Buddha, who lived over 2,000 years ago. He was born into one of the richest and most powerful royal families in India and spent the first twenty-nine years of his life living as a prince. However, despite having all the health, wealth, and good relationships he could wish for, he still felt incomplete, and he could also see a great need in others for a real solution to life's problems. Finally he came to understand that most people look for happiness in the wrong place! He felt sure that true, lasting happiness could be found simply by understanding and developing the mind.

He decided to give up his inheritance and devote the rest of his life to attaining the ultimate state of wisdom and happiness, so that he could share this with others. All of Buddha's teachings were recorded and passed down, and to this day we have a pure, unbroken lineage of the path to full enlightenment. This lineage is now firmly established in the West. We do not have to travel far to find it.

New Kadampa Tradition

One of the largest international Buddhist organizations is the New Kadampa Tradition (NKT). Established in 1976 by Tibetan meditation master, Geshe Kelsang Gyatso Rinpoche, its purpose is "to present the mainstream of Buddhist teachings in a way that is relevant and immediately applicable to the contemporary Western way of life." Most cities and towns in the UK have an NKT residential center or meditation group and many others are opening in the U.S., Europe, and all over the world. (See appendix 3 for books by Geshe Kelsang Gyatso on Buddhism and Buddhist practice.)

To find your nearest Buddhist center, or if you would like a teacher to give an introductory talk on Buddhism in your area, contact one of the following organizations:

UK Contact:
New Kadampa Tradition
Conishead Priory
Ulverston, Cumbria, LA12 9QQ
England

Phone/fax: 01229 588533 (within UK)
E-mail: kadampa@dircon.co.uk
Internet: www.kadampa.org

U.S. Contact:
New Kadampa Tradition
Kadampa Meditation Center
47 Sweeney Road
PO Box 447
Glen Spey, NY 12737

Phone: 845-856-9000
Toll-free: 1-877-KADAMPA (1-877-523-2672)
E-mail: KadampaCenter@aol.com
Internet: www.kadampa.org

International Temples Project
"Building for World Peace"
www.kadampa.org

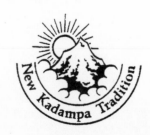

Appendix 3:
Books on Buddhism

The following list of books are good for beginners as well as more experienced practitioners. All are written by Geshe Kelsang Gyatso.

Gyatso, Geshe Kelsang. *Eight Steps To Happiness: The Buddhist Way of Loving Kindness.* United Kingdom: Tharpa Publications, 2000.

_____. *Introduction to Buddhism: An Explanation of the Buddhist Way of Life.* United Kingdom: Tharpa Publications, 1993.

_____. *Joyful Path of Good Fortune: The Complete Buddhist Path to Enlightenment.* United Kingdom: Tharpa Publications, 1996.

_____. *Meaningful To Behold: The Bodhisattva's Way of Life.* United Kingdom: Tharpa Publications, 1998.

_____. *The Meditation Handbook: A Practical Guide to Meditation*. United Kingdom: Tharpa Publications, 1995.

_____. *Transform Your Life: A Blissful Journey*. United Kingdom: Tharpa Publications, 2001.

_____. *Universal Compassion: Transforming Your Life through Love and Compassion*. United Kingdom: Tharpa Publications, 1997.

Appendix 4:
Hypothyroidism

(*The following information continues from Gina Wright's contributing story, "Low Thyroid Function," on pages 153–154.*)

Thyroid function blood tests, or TFTs as doctors call them, have a very wide reference range. Thyroid stimulating hormone (TSH), as produced by your pituitary to make the thyroid work harder (hence, my throbbing big toe), can be considered normal in the range of 0.5–6.0 and anything in between; even borderline is classified as normal.

T4 (thyroxine) can range from 60–140 and, again, is classified as normal if you are within its scale of reference, despite any symptoms you may have. If your blood is "okay," you are told you are fine. "The symptoms are in your head, go away, and pull yourself together," is a typical doctor's response. The problem also is that although your blood tests look brilliant, your body is not converting the thyroxine into a form your body can use (this is called T3). Very few doctors or hospitals are willing to test for this, yet it is vitally important to know what your body is doing and if it is benefiting from the amount of thyroxine floating around.

Are you one of these people? If so, don't despair. I have discovered that there are doctors who listen to you and your symptoms. Blood tests are not everything, and there is help out there. One of the easiest and most accurate ways of diagnosing low thyroid function is the Barnes Basal Temperature Test. This test, championed by Dr. Broda Barnes, proves low thyroid function by the running temperature of your body. It's easy to do and all you need is a thermometer. For women, it should be carried out on the fifth day of your menstrual cycle for four days, unless you no longer have periods. For men, the test can be done anytime.

Place the thermometer under your arm first thing in the morning before you get out of bed. Leave it there for ten minutes and then take the reading. If your temperature is consistently below 37 degrees Celsius or 98.6 degrees Fahrenheit, then you have low thyroid function. I was 35.5 degrees Celsius—no wonder I was always freezing!

My doctor knew I had a problem, but to go against blood tests and "buck the system" was too big of a step. He didn't know what to do or where to send me. The chances are your own doctor will feel the same way unless you change his or her view by making the doctor listen to you and to take notice of the thousands of patients who are suffering because of poor interpretations of thyroid blood tests.

There are over sixty symptoms of low thyroid function. Here are some of them:

- Weight gain or loss
- Digestive problems and constipation
- Low body temperature, feeling cold all the time
- Tiredness and weakness
- Brain fog (feeling like your head is stuffed with cotton)
- Poor memory, lack of concentration
- Slow pulse and low blood pressure
- High cholesterol
- Hair, skin, and nail problems
- Low, husky voice
- Muscle and joint pains (low thyroid function is now being linked to chronic fatigue syndrome)
- Menstrual changes or fertility problems
- Depression, change in mood
- Low self-esteem, lack of confidence
- Lack of interest in normal activities
- Low sex drive
- Eye problems, e.g., gritty eyes, sensitivity to light, dryness, blurriness
- Neck and throat complaints, e.g., discomfort with clothing around the neck, difficulty swallowing, a choking feeling, as if something is stuck in the throat

- Hearing/tinnitus
- More infections and lowered immune resistance
- Allergies
- Sleep apnea and snoring
- Breathing difficulties, asthma-like symptoms
- Dizziness, vertigo
- Puffiness, swelling

If you would like to exercise patient power, be informed and make a difference to thyroid treatment by joining the Thyroid Support Association UK. We'll make a stand for sufferers everywhere.

Gina Wright

Publisher's note: If you would like to contact Gina Wright, please visit Llewellyn.com for a link to the author's website, or write to the author in care of Llewellyn Publications.

Bibliography

Bach, Edward. *Heal Thyself*. England: C.W. Daniel Co., Ltd., 1931.

Byers, Dwight. *Better Health with Foot Reflexology*. Ingham Publishing.

De Vries, Jan. *Body Energy*. Mainstream Publishing.

Dougans, Inge. *Reflexology: A Practical Introduction*. Element Books.

Ingham, Eunice. *Stories the Feet Can Tell Through Reflexology*. Ingham Publishing.

———. *Stories the Feet Have Told Through Reflexology*. Ingham Publishing.

Kunz, Kevin and Barbara. *The Complete Guide to Foot Reflexology*. Thorssons.

Stormer, Chris. *Reflexology*. Hodder and Stoughton.

Index

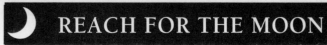
REACH FOR THE MOON

Llewellyn publishes hundreds of books on your favorite subjects! To get these exciting books, including the ones on the following pages, check your local bookstore or order them directly from Llewellyn.

Order by Phone
- Call toll-free within the U.S. and Canada, 1-800-THE MOON
- In Minnesota, call (651) 291-1970
- We accept VISA, MasterCard, and American Express

Order by Mail
- Send the full price of your order (MN residents add 7% sales tax) in U.S. funds, plus postage & handling to:

  Llewellyn Worldwide
  P.O. Box 64383, Dept. 0-7387-0098-3
  St. Paul, MN 55164–0383, U.S.A.

Postage & Handling
- **Standard** (U.S., Mexico, & Canada)

If your order is:

  $20.00 or under, add $5.00
  $20.01–$100.00, add $6.00
  Over $100, shipping is free

(Continental U.S. orders ship UPS. AK, HI, PR, & P.O. Boxes ship USPS 1st class. Mex. & Can. ship PMB.)

- **Second Day Air** (Continental U.S. only): $10.00 for one book + $1.00 per each additional book
- **Express** (AK, HI, & PR only) [Not available for P.O. Box delivery. For street address delivery only.]: $15.00 for one book + $1.00 per each additional book
- **International Surface Mail:** Add $1.00 per item
- **International Airmail:** Books—Add the retail price of each item; Non-book items—Add $5.00 per item

  Please allow 4–6 weeks for delivery on all orders.
  Postage and handling rates subject to change.

Discounts
We offer a 20% discount to group leaders or agents. You must order a minimum of 5 copies of the same book to get our special quantity price.

FREE CATALOG

Get a free copy of our color catalog, *New Worlds of Mind and Spirit*. Subscribe for just $10.00 in the United States and Canada ($30.00 overseas, airmail). Many bookstores carry *New Worlds*—ask for it!

Visit our website at www.llewellyn.com for more information.

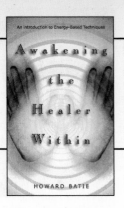

Awakening the Healer Within

HOWARD BATIE

If you are looking into alternative methods of healing, you have a growing and often bewildering selection to choose from. Which healing modalities are recommended for specific ailments, and do they really work? *Awakening the Healer Within* discusses several energy-based healing techniques that have repeatedly demonstrated a positive effect on clients.

The root cause of physical disease is contained in the faulty patterns in the etheric body (the aura) or higher energy bodies (emotional, mental, and spiritual). Healing work that is performed on these energy levels can often keep disease from manifesting on the physical level.

This book discusses significant modalities for all levels of your being: physical (healing touch and reiki), etheric (spiritual surgery and reflective healing), emotional and mental (rohun and hypnotherapy), and spiritual (light energization).

1-56718-055-8
216 pp., 6 x 9 $12.95

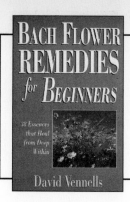

Bach Flower Remedies for Beginners

38 Essences that Heal from Deep Within

DAVID F. VENNELLS

Here is a system of healing that is natural, powerful, and simple to use. If you can observe someone's state of mind, you can select the appropriate Bach Flower Remedy for that person. Someone who is always impatient and quick in thought, for example, might need Impatiens. Someone who is dreamy and needs a lot of sleep may be a classic Clematis.

Bach Flower Remedies work on the subtle mental and emotional levels of the mind, where illness actually begins. They target the particular negative states of mind that give rise to physical symptoms, thus protecting us from future illness.

- Read the story of Dr. Edward Bach, the man who discovered this system of healing
- Learn how the remedies actually work to activate and support the healing process
- Prepare your own remedies
- Learn how to prescribe the remedies for anyone, including children and pets
- Refer to the dictionary of 38 remedies with detailed analysis of the main mental and emotional symptoms

0-7387-0047-9, 312 pp., 5³⁄₁₆ x 6 $12.95
Available in Spanish.

To order, call 1-800-THE MOON
Prices subject to change without notice

Reiki for Beginners
Mastering Natural Healing Techniques

DAVID F. VENNELLS

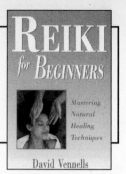

Reiki is a simple yet profound system of hands-on healing developed in Japan during the 1800s. Millions of people worldwide have already benefited from its peaceful healing intelligence that transcends cultural and religious boundaries. It can have a profound effect on health and well-being by rebalancing, cleansing, and renewing your internal energy system.

Reiki for Beginners gives you the very basic and practical principles of using Reiki as a simple healing technique, as well as its more deeply spiritual aspects as a tool for personal growth and self-awareness. Unravel your inner mysteries, heal your wounds, and discover your potential for great happiness. Follow the history of Reiki, from founder Dr. Mikao Usui's search for a universal healing technique, to the current development of a global Reiki community. Also included are many new ideas, techniques, advice, philosophies, contemplations, and meditations that you can use to deepen and enhance your practice.

1-56718-767-6
264 pp., 5³⁄₁₆ x 8, illus. $12.95
Available in Spanish.